Shiatsu for Lovers

NATHAN B. STRAUSS

The healing art of Shiatsu, as it developed in Japan, involves close contact between the giver and the receiver, as is the case with most Japanese massage techniques. It is no wonder that the art of loving massage, *Shiatsu for Lovers*, developed and became so successful in Japan.

Shiatsu for Lovers enables lovers to maximize their physical pleasure by massaging and manipulating the areas and points in each other's bodies that enhance and arouse passion. Knowledge of these points, and treating them lovingly with Shiatsu, will lead the couple to new heights of ecstasy.

Nathan B. Strauss, who lives in New York and is a physiotherapist, specializes in alternative healing methods such as reflexology and Shiatsu.

Shiatsu for Lovers

A Practical Guide

Nathan B. Strauss

Astrolog Publishing House

Astrolog Publishing House
P. O. Box 1123, Hod Hasharon 45111, Israel
Tel: 972-9-7412044
Fax: 972-9-7442714
E-Mail: info@astrolog.co.il
Astrolog Web Site: www.astrolog.co.il

ISBN 965-494-091-4

Published by Astrolog Publishing House 2000

Printed in Israel
1 3 5 7 9 10 8 6 4 2

CONTENTS

* **The meridians**
* **The effect of Shiatsu touch**
* **The massage action on the body**
* **The principles of Shiatsu pressure, massage. and acupuncture**
* **Basic ethics**
* **The basic pressure methods in a Shiatsu treatment**
Vertical pressure - Stationary pressure - Equal pressure - Supporting pressure
* **Massage techniques**
Effleurage - Kneading - Squeezing (petrissage) - Revolving - Rolling - Rubbing-pulling - Turning-rubbing - Pulling pressure - Shaking - Tapping with the fingers - Tapping with cupped hands - Slapping movement - Chopping - Pulling the nape and hair - Shampooing - Neuromuscular massage on both sides of the spinal column - Feathering
* **Essential points**
The "Intersection of the Three Yins" point - The "Sea of Blood" point - The "Original Chi" point - The "Walking Three Miles" point - The "Pass Organ" point - The "Middle Extreme" point - The "Crooked Bone" point - The "Conception Vessel One" point - The pressure point below the knee - The pressure point at the base of the calf - The pressure point on the outer side of the calf - The pressure point above the knee - The pressure point on the outer side of the thigh - The pressure point at the top of the

bridge of the nose - The pressure point on the sole of the
foot - The stomach meridian pressure points - The liver
meridian pressure point - The spleen meridian pressure
points - The pressure points on the back - The pressure
points on the upper thigh - The pressure points on the ear -
The pressure points on the hand - The pressure points
between the eyebrows - The pressure points between the
upper lip and the nose
  * **A massage using oils and essential oils**
  * **Sexually arousing oils**
  * **Preparation and method of massage**
  * **Advice for the massage**
  * **A massage for sexual arousal, combined with Shiatsu**
pressures

2. Shiatsu for Lovers   112

  * **Unique pressure techniques in Shiatsu for Lovers**
Thumb pressure - Finger pressure - "Pinching" pressure -
Pressure using the pads of the hand
  * **Problems, diseases, and treatment situations**
Relieving menstrual cramps and pains
Points for relieving menopausal symptoms
Points for relieving mid-life symptoms in men
Frigidity
Preferred sexual arousal points
"Distant" points for treating sexual problems
The Love Points - points that are "close"
Points for relieving extreme tension

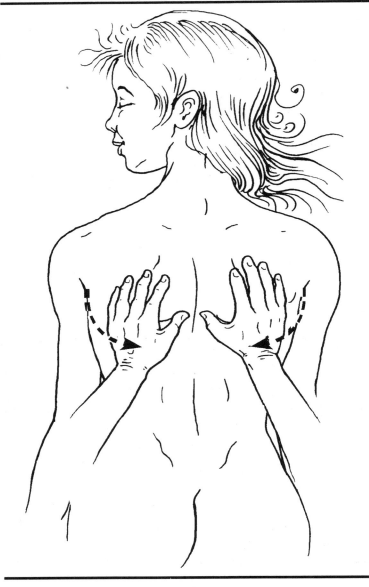

1

Introduction

"Shiatsu" is a Japanese word meaning "finger pressure." "Shi" means "finger" in Japanese, while "atsu" means "pressure." Shiatsu is essentially a manual therapy that applies static pressure to various points and lines on the surface of the body. The points are called "acu points" or "tsubo points," and are also used in acupuncture.

The lines along which the points are located are called "meridians." The concepts of points and lines can be found in various eastern arts, and throughout Chinese and Japanese medicine.

The theories behind all of these healing methods - herbal medicine, Shiatsu, acupuncture, acupressure, and so on - are almost all based on curing the disease, the problem, or the imbalance by means of the patient's own natural healing energies.

According to eastern medicine, man and nature are one. We are what we eat, drink, and live by. When we lose the natural balance and harmony between us and nature (a state of balance is the optimal one), a disease occurs.

In fact, the healer is simply an "intermediary" who stimulates the life energy - the "Chi" or the "Ki" - of the patient, using medicinal herbs, acupuncture, or pressure on various points and energy-flow lines (meridians). The aim is to restore the patient's energy flow to its natural and harmonious course by releasing the mental or physical blockages that disrupt it, and ultimately lead to a state of disease, which serves as a warning of an imbalance in the body. The disease itself is not actually the problem. Like an alarm bell or a red light, it "informs" us that the body is not in a state of balance.

For this reason, the treatment does not necessarily focus on the disease or the problem, but on the patient himself. The healer matches his healing work - or more precisely, the stimulation of the energy - to the patient's life energy, in order to restore harmony between the patient and nature, and to stimulate his self-healing power and his life energy.

In accordance with this approach, the diagnosis is made, and treatment administered, by means of the hands, without the use of any instruments. Moxas, the needles used in acupuncture, and various implements, are not considered "instruments" or "appliances." Their purpose is not to penetrate the body with "something new" that did not exist there previously, but rather simply to stimulate the body's self-healing powers, in order to restore energetic balance and the correct flow of life force in the meridians. The same is true for the use of medicinal herbs, and by healing via correct nutrition and eating, according to the person's condition. Food and medicinal herbs are not substances that are foreign to the body, but consist of the same components that make up our body, since the food we eat serves to build up our body, and constitutes the general raw material of our body.

In Shiatsu, we work on the meridians, in which the life force - Chi - flows.

*

In Shiatsu for Lovers, we concentrate on the meridians (and on certain points on them) that are highly effective in the realms of love, sex, and harmony within couples. However, before focusing on Shiatsu for Lovers, we must become better acquainted with the basic principles that form the foundation of Shiatsu, and the fundamentals of massage (including massage with essential oils).

The meridians

The meridians are energy paths. In our bodies, there are many "paths" of different types. There are paths that convey nervous impulses (neurotransmitters), there are paths that convey blood and particles of food, and so on. It will be easier for us to imagine the meridians, which are invisible energetic paths, if we compare their action to the way in which the blood circulates through our bodies in the veins, arteries, and capillaries, or the way in which the neurotransmitters travel along the nerves throughout our bodies. The difference is that the meridians are paths that convey energy and vital force (Chi). They can be described as a system that is similar to the nervous system, but more delicate and less tangible. Here we have to clarify a point that is essential for proceeding with our reading and understanding. Every organism in the universe, as well as the universe itself, consists of many different layers, some of them "thicker" - that is, more concrete, more "substantial" and perceivable by our physical senses, and some of them "thinner" - more delicate, and not always visible or perceivable by our "ordinary" senses. The meridians constitute a more delicate parallel of the body's circulatory system. The circulatory system is more concrete, and its channels can be seen with the naked eye, and felt physically; the nervous system is "thinner" and more delicate, so that we need a microscope to discern its small, thin parts, and an electron microscope to discern particles such as neurotransmitters that pass through it. The meridian network is even finer, but instruments that will enable us to discern it are being developed.

The meridian network consists of numerous paths that run the length and breadth of the body, and, just like the nervous system, where there are main nerve centers, there are meridian points that constitute energy centers at the intersections of the paths.

According to Chinese medicine, there are numerous paths and sub-paths, but only 26 main paths (12 pairs on either side of the body and two single paths). Those are the ones used in Shiatsu and Chinese acupuncture. Chi - life energy - flows along the meridians, and from there to the spinal cord, the nerves, and millions of tiny energy-conveying paths. The spinal cord is considered to be the main axis around which electro-magnetic energy exists. The northern pole of human energy is located at the "base" of the brain (just before the beginning of the first neck vertebra), and the southern pole is located at the tip of the spinal column. Since the energy paths flow in a parallel manner, there is an interactive relationship between them, in which they reinforce and energize one another. This increases the strength of the electro-magnetic field. In order to preserve this process of mutual reinforcement and energizing, the flows of energies must be normal and harmonious.

In order to understand the creation of a harmonious or a disharmonious state, we must take into account the factors that we have already mentioned: the importance of the state of harmony between body, mind, and spirit, as well as the system of constant energetic links between us, our surroundings, and nature, and between us and the universal energy. This energetic system is operated by the person's awareness, just as we activate our thoughts and feelings. It links the body, mind, and spirit, and is activated by the person's life energy, which controls and understands his life with the help of and by means of his awareness. When we are in a state of spiritual harmony with the universe, we attain a harmonious flow in our body, mind, and spirit, and our electro-magnetic field increases accordingly.

By means of massage, Shiatsu, and various healing techniques, we can release energetic barriers that are liable to occur in this system, balance situations of lack in the system, or states of blockage.

What is the life force that flows in the meridians? Life force, which is also called Chi, Ki, Prana, and other names, is the dynamic (active, creative) force that gives the body life. It is the force that guards every part of the organism and ensures its harmonious and balanced functioning.

In western medicine, the life force is called "homeostasis." Examples of homeostatic mechanisms in the body are: (a) body temperature, which the body balances according to the surroundings and internal needs by means of a number of balance mechanisms; and (b) the pH balance (acid-base) - the body normally tends slightly toward base. In an abnormal situation, the body activates a number of mechanisms in order to restore balance, via the respiratory and metabolic systems (for example, by means of the kidneys). When there is too much acidity, the condition can be balanced via the respiratory system - the body will secrete more carbon dioxide - and via the metabolic system - the kidneys will recycle base molecules, and, of course, vice versa.

One of the aims of the Shiatsu massage is to reinforce and sharpen the life force and the natural, correct flow of the meridians, while we release and open energy blockages, and balance conditions of excess and of lack. Of course, restoring the body's balance does not occur merely on the physical level, but also on the emotional-mental and spiritual level.

The effect of Shiatsu touch

The advantages of treatment with Shiatsu touch - especially Shiatsu for Lovers - are numerous. It constitutes an effective mode of treatment that helps the patient achieve optimal balance and health. First and foremost, Shiatsu touch stimulates the movement of Chi - the life force, and the energy - in the patient's body. This is the first procedure we use in order to help the patient recover and get him into a state of optimal health. It helps stimulate the movement of the blood, and improves blood circulation. Its effect on the nervous system is major; it helps to calm or stimulate it, according to what is needed and intended, and in this way, together with the influence of the muscular system, significantly helps the patient attain a state of physical and mental tranquillity, and is instrumental in reducing stress and releasing tension. In addition, Shiatsu touch induces a state of emotional and physiological stability in the patient, and helps him attain physical awareness, which permits him to "understand" his body and become more familiar with it.

By means of this mechanism, Shiatsu reinforces both body and soul. Naturally, when we combine massage with Shiatsu (which focuses on exerting *pressure* on the points), we get a Shiatsu massage whose advantages are manifold.

Specifically, Shiatsu massage is wonderful for treating various back problems, muscular spasms, stiffness of the body and of the joints; it helps increase the flexibility of the body and of the joints, alleviates various pains such as headaches, stomach-aches, pains in the shoulders, a stiff neck, and so on, and provides relief from menstrual problems.

In other words, Shiatsu - not only in the form of Shiatsu for Lovers - is good for treating about 40 percent of the causes of problems and malfunctioning in an active sex life. In addition, Shiatsu improves the flow of blood, which is responsible for causing 25 percent of the problems in sex. The importance of Shiatsu for Lovers lies in the fact that it focuses on the sexual system, and is effective in solving about 90 percent of the problems that occur in it. Shiatsu is also excellent for relieving pains and solving problems that derive from strenuous work, athletic activity, and other activities that exhaust the body in one way or another. Since Shiatsu massage improves the general flow in the body - the flow of blood and the flow of energy, releases energetic and physical blockages, and stimulates Chi - life force, it is a wonderful technique for preventing many common diseases. In this way, it also fortifies the immune system, causing the patient to feel generally calmer in his daily life, and much better physically.

The massage action on the body

Many people are familiar with the wonderful physical feeling after a refreshing and healthy massage. Stiff muscles relax, painful areas hurt less, and one's general feeling improves. Massage has a beneficial effect on blood circulation, and on the cleansing and excretion of the toxins from our body; in this way, it affects our entire body.

A very important aspect that massage addresses is the reduction of stress. Since the physical actions of massage are better known, and are also felt in an immediate and tangible way directly after the treatment, we will concentrate on the effect of stress reduction, which is a cumulative effect, all of whose facets are not manifested immediately (except, of course, the good psychological feeling that follows the massage directly). Stress reduction is immensely important for the person's entire mental and physical health, and especially for the quality of his love relationships and sex life. In past years, stress was not related to terribly seriously, and the importance of stress reduction was not high on the list of priorities. Today, many practitioners, physicians, and researchers have reached the conclusion that one of the main causes of damage to the immune system, as well as to the functions of the body as a whole, is stress.

Stress, or tension, is a well-known and common concept in contemporary achievement-oriented society. The daily stresses to which people are subjected are enormous, and the possibility of finding oneself in situations of tension or stress exists in the workplace, on the highways, at home - in fact, almost everywhere. Stress, or tension, is essentially a physical phenomenon that is controlled by the nervous system. The emotional process that causes stress triggers physical, nervous, and hormonal mechanisms. Constantly being in situations of stress and tension exhausts the body as a result of the repeated and persistent activation of these mechanisms, which, from an evolutionary point of view, were meant to serve us in life-threatening situations, so as to make our attack or escape action more effective. Today, however, they are triggered over and over again in many people throughout the day. Situations such as falling behind schedule at work, domestic disputes, study pressures, excessive demands from children, driving, financial pressures, and so on, all create tension, and gradually undermine all the body's systems.

In one way or another, every holistic therapy, as well as Eastern healing methods, concerns the idea of reducing stress and tension so as to improve the general condition of the patient. It is amazing to what extent a treatment that helps reduce the patient's level of stress is likely to help him in every aspect of life, while fortifying him mentally and physically, and diverting the energies that were invested in the stress factors and in coping with them to useful and beneficial channels.

Being in a constant state of stress is liable to exhaust the person mentally and physically, and to expose and cause various diseases. It is well-known that there are many diseases whose correlation to the patient's level of stress is direct and obvious. Other diseases are rendered considerably more serious by stress and tension. Among the diseases that are known to have a high correlation to psychological stress are asthma, various menstrual disorders, problems of the immune system (high susceptibility to infections, and so on), hypertension, ulcers, diabetes, rheumatoid arthritis, colitis, headaches and migraines, cancer, heart diseases, blood vessel disorders, psoriasis, and many other maladies; as well as, of course, problems such as impotence, frigidity, vaginismus, premature ejaculation, and other problems linked to sexual intercourse and the relationship between the members of a couple.

Massage, and even more so, massage with essential oils, plays an effective and significant role in reducing stress. People who are under constant stress (and that, of course, is a subjective feeling), who suffer from a huge workload, from keeping to a tight schedule, and so on, require massage on a regular basis - at least once or twice a week - in order to avoid future stress-caused damage to their bodies. Sometimes people wonder how it is possible that a 50-year-old person who does not smoke, who eats healthy food, and who even jogs along the shore twice a week, has a heart attack. This question forgets to relate to the cumulative situations of stress that the person experienced during the course of his life - situations that have a high probability of leaving their mark on his body's systems many years later.

We must remember that every physical disease has a psychological aspect. Frequently, the disease is an expression of various mental processes - conscious or unconscious. We have to know how to identify them and use Shiatsu to liberate the soul and release the emotional blockages that are causing the stagnation. When we treat the psychological aspect, we enable the life energy to flow more easily, and in that way help the body to recover.

Often, we can discern a chain of negative events that causes the disease, whether on the mental or physical level; in most cases, we discover that the situation is flawed in both. For example, the chain of negative events is liable to start with a situation of stress or trauma that causes the person to develop a negative attitude toward life or toward a particular situation. The negative attitude, a lack of confidence in life, constitutes the most widespread reason for sleeplessness and insomnia. When the person has difficulty falling asleep because of a high level of stress, fear of tomorrow, or the inability to wind down and relax, fatigue accumulates and leaves its mark on him; he feels too exhausted to participate in any physical activity - even simple walking. He tries to balance his state of fatigue with food, coffee, or other stimulants, and begins to feel heavy and listless because of a vicious circle that has been created.

When anxiety, depression, existential fears, financial worries, or anxiety about the family are added, the sleep problems are exacerbated, and at the same time, the physiological and immune systems are undermined. The action of the nervous system becomes unbalanced when the immune system is weakened. The person experiences an overall bad feeling, for which he tries to compensate by smoking, drinking too much "stimulating" coffee, eating irregularly, and so on. This situation is liable to culminate in the neglect of environmental, physical, and mental hygiene, which, of course, aggravates the emotional problems. The person is liable to feel listless at this stage, and he does not feel like doing various things, having a good time, or seeing people; he locks himself up even more in the vicious circle.

When we add to the chain of negative events a situation of physical weakness in one of the body's systems, hormonal problems or a lack of hormonal balance, as well as menopause, PMS, or other tiresome premenstrual symptoms, we get an even heavier load.

In situations of a lack of physical or mental balance such as these, a disease or a problem is liable to occur in one of the person's body systems, generally in the one that is weakest in that person. For instance, when the immune system is vulnerable, viral and bacterial diseases occur. Unfortunately, most people discern the formation of the psycho-physical chain of negative events only after the occurrence of the disease in a body system that was unable to withstand the load. When we discern the chain of negative events, we often discover pressure, tension or various states of emotional or mental imbalance in one of its primary links.

In most of the sexual problems described in this book, there is a primary link that includes situations of stress. In these cases, which are so widespread, our first aim is to induce a state of calmness and relaxation in the patient. Massage is one of the most marvelous ways of relieving the burden, and constitutes one of the first steps toward breaking the chain of negative events.

When we set about treating a person who suffers from a chain of negative events such as the one described above, we must pay attention to his nutritional state, and watch out for nutrients that are lacking, an inadequate daily diet, the consumption of unsuitable foods, or the abuse of stimulants such as caffeine; all this must be exchanged for healthy, fortifying foods. Appropriate, healthy, physical activity is also a necessary or effective stage in a full treatment of the person. Moreover, we have to draw the person's attention to his attitude toward life. A depressed, angry, bitter attitude is not in the least helpful in breaking the chain of negative events.

During massage, when we help the person to feel calm and relaxed, we enable his body and mind to rest and begin the process of self-balancing and accumulating energy and renewed strength. The renewal of the energy supplies will lead to improved activity during the day, to an increase in the level of general motivation, and the motivation for self-treatment (which is very important when there is a need for a program of physical activity, nutritional changes, diet, and so on), and better and more satisfactory sleep. Better sleep enhances the body's healing powers, helps change the person's attitude toward his surroundings, creates a generally better and calmer feeling, and reduces the level of daily stress, nervousness, and pressure. When the person's mood is good, his motivation to balance his mental and physical condition increases and strengthens, and he is able to cope with problems and tasks in a calm, effective, and stress-free way. There is even an increase in his motivation to make nutritional changes, as well as to engage in physical activity, in outdoor activities, in hobbies, and in anything that is likely to make him feel better and healthier.

When the person permits himself to enjoy the beneficial pleasures of life, eats correctly, and engages in physical activity, he gains a healthier and more pliant body, and a calmer and more balanced mind. All these, along with the reduction of daily stress levels, especially by means of Shiatsu massage on a regular basis of at least once or twice a week, strengthen the immune system and the body's healing powers. Together with the person's efforts and personal motivation to improve his lifestyle, habits, and general attitude toward life, we significantly increase his chances to recover and fully regain his health.

Here I will add that the aspect of life in which we see the most significant change is in the realm of sex and love (and on the physical plane, the most significant improvement is in blood pressure). Therefore, when we want to effect a change in the realm of love and sex, we will focus on massaging the points for Shiatsu for Lovers (to be discussed).

The principles of Shiatsu pressure, massage, and acupuncture

During the many years that teachers and practitioners of Shiatsu, acupuncture, massage, and healers who healed by means of touch practiced their arts, a number of touch, pressure, and massage methods formed, and they were found to be especially effective.

We will present several methods of pressure and touch that are easy to apply, and have a beneficial effect on body and mind. Some of them were developed and discovered by Shiatsu practitioners, others by acupressure and massage experts.

In Shiatsu massage, creativity, intuition, the practitioner's feeling when touching the patient, and the patient's feeling - the type of touch that is pleasant for him, the strength, intensity, and depth - these are the things that must guide the practitioner, professional or amateur, along his path of treatment. These principles must be remembered when we administer self-treatment.

It is highly recommended that we try out the various pressure techniques on our own bodies before treating someone else. In this way, we become acquainted with the character of the different forms of pressure and massage, their action, and their effect on mind and body. Trying it out on ourselves is one of the best ways for the practitioner to achieve a deeper, more sensitive and more aware feeling of the patient's body.

When we set out to administer treatment using touch, pressure, and massage, we have to remember an extremely important rule. The more the pressure derives from a stronger "source of strength" in the practitioner, the less strength it will require from the practitioner's body. That is, when pressure is applied by the hands only, it is necessary to press more forcefully, since only the muscles of the hands are activated. This demands a lot more strength, and is liable to exhaust or wear the practitioner out quickly. Moreover, it produces pressure that is less steady and even. In contrast, when we use the weight of our body, and the pressure derives from the base of the body - the pelvis, which is the powerful point of balance of the body, especially when the patient is lying on the floor, or when he is lying on a massage bed at a height that is right for the practitioner, pressure can be applied to the patient's body far more effectively. It is possible to apply pressure, which ultimately emanates from the practitioner's hands, using the shoulder muscles, the abdominal region, and the pelvis, and even use the body weight in a suitable way, taking care not to weigh too heavily on the patient, in order to create the desired pressure on the patient's body.

Even when we only use our fingers to apply pressure to Shiatsu points, it is important to notice from which source or muscle system we are applying the pressure, and find the position in which we can apply the steadiest and most balanced pressure that does not tire the body parts that perform the massage and apply the pressure.

It is very important to be aware of the patient's physical structure and condition. If he is thin, slender, weak, fragile, or particularly sensitive, we apply light, delicate pressure. This is extremely important when treating the elderly and children. The best way is to be aware and to listen to the patient's body. No less important is listening to his opinion - asking him how he feels, and if the pressure is appropriate, correct, and pleasant for him. Similarly, when we treat bigger, stronger, or heavier people, we may have to apply more pressure. Of course, we listen to the patient's body.

When the pressure is too strong, it is sometimes possible to discern a slight contraction, which expresses a certain resistance. This resistance is likely to occur for a number of reasons, some of which are unique to the patient. Before we describe the methods of pressure, massage, and touch, we will explain a number of reasons that are liable to engender resistance to touch. Some of them are seemingly very simple, and others are more complex, but ultimately all of them have the same effect. When the patient reacts to the practitioner's touch with resistance, or with a "contraction," it means that there is a serious glitch in the course of the treatment. In such a case, the effectiveness of the treatment diminishes. The greater the resistance, the less effective the treatment.

Cold hands: When the practitioner's hands are cold, and he places them on the patient's exposed body, the patient's body immediately and naturally contracts as a result of the cold touch. This contraction, of course, contradicts one of the main principles of massage - the relaxing and calming of the patient's body. A situation like this must under no circumstances be permitted to arise. Before touching the patient's body, it is important that for the practitioner first warm his hands.

A cold room, or a generally cold feeling: This situation is also liable to make the patient's body contract. Feelings of warmth or cold are individual. There are patients who are less sensitive to cold, and those who are more sensitive. In any event, during the massage, especially when the body is partially or entirely exposed, the feeling of cold is liable to make the patient's body contract in a way that makes the practitioner's work very difficult (even if he is not aware of it or does not feel it!). In addition, inner tremors are likely to occur, and these detract from the effectiveness of the treatment and distract the patient from the treatment, and the healing. Moreover, they greatly impair the body's ability to relax and calm down, as well as the patient's ability to succumb to mental tranquillity - factors that are extremely important for the effectiveness of the treatment and the reduction of stress.

For this reason, it is very important to see that the room is heated prior to the treatment during fall or winter, or in the evening, when it is cooler. Under no circumstances must there be an open window through which wind can blow onto the patient, when his body is exposed, unless it is summer, and the weather is hot, and the wind is light and gentle, and not direct.

It is very important to ensure that any part of the patient's body that is not being treated is covered. Not only is this important for preventing colds or a feeling of cold in the exposed body, but it prevents the patient from feeling uncomfortable. When one of the parts of his body is exposed and naked, but the practitioner is touching, massaging, supporting, or warming it, the feeling of nakedness should not bother the patient (unless he has some kind of problem with touch and exposure, and that is quite a different story). In contrast, an exposed body part that is not being treated is quite naturally liable to cause the patient to experience a feeling of unpleasant exposure and discomfort.

In Shiatsu for Lovers or an erotic massage, which is performed by couples, the attitude toward exposed body parts that are not being touched at that moment is quite different, since the ultimate aim of the massage - besides, of course, soothing and relaxing the body - is different. Generally speaking, it is a matter of two people who are more open to each other from the point of view of the desire for touch, as well as the acknowledged aim of the massage.

In order to prevent a situation of an exposed and cold body part, every part that is not being treated or massaged should be covered with a towel or a light blanket. Moreover, after we have finished massaging a particular part, it should be covered immediately with a towel (or a blanket in winter) in order to prevent the muscles that have just undergone a process of soothing and relaxing from becoming chilled, and to ensure that the inner warming of the body continues the effect caused by the touch and massage.

Pressure that is too strong: In various methods of treatment, including Shiatsu, the practitioner uses the weight of his body in order to create even, deep, and significant pressure on the patient's tissues. Care must be taken to ensure that the pressure is not too strong, because if it is painful, it is liable to disrupt the course of the treatment. In massage, pressure that is too strong, or "penetration" that is too fast into the patient's tissues by the fingers, especially into a place that has been stiff for a long time, is liable to achieve the opposite effect. The patient's body is liable to manifest resistance to the invasive touch, and to contract even more, thus making the practitioner's work harder. For this reason, it is of cardinal importance to "listen" to the patient's body and to pay true and focused attention to his responses to touch.

Superficial pressure, pressure that is too light, gentle, or ticklish: Fluttering movements of the fingertips and a gentle movement of stroking or even of light tickling are suitable and pleasant during a massage whose aim is sexual arousal;

however, during a therapeutic massage, they are liable to create an unpleasant feeling in the patient by stimulating his nerve endings in an annoying way. In a therapeutic massage, it is very important that the movement be steady and of the correct strength. Sometimes, when the pressure is too weak, the patient feels that the pressure is insufficient, and he yearns for a more substantial pressure. As a result, his feeling of relaxation and tranquillity are liable to be undermined. For this reason, it is important to ensure that the pressure is not too weak. We must not be diffident about asking a person whose body and needs we do not yet know very well if the pressure is too gentle, too strong, or suitable, and request that he tell us if he wants stronger or weaker pressure.

Long nails: In therapeutic massage, long nails can only be a nuisance. While there are experienced and professional practitioners - mainly women - who over the years have learned various ways of administering treatment without cutting their nails, uncut nails significantly limit the practitioner, since he is unable to perform many techniques without hurting the patient. When a finger has to penetrate deep tissues, an uncut nail will leave a red mark on the patient's body, and is liable to hurt or scratch him. The same goes for the squeezing technique - and other techniques - in which long nails get in the way and are liable to scratch the patient's body. A person who wants to perform a perfect, professional, and enjoyable massage, without any disruptions, would do well to cut his nails. Of course, nails can scratch the patient's body by mistake at any point; this is not pleasant, and causes the patient's body to resist the touch quickly and intensely. In Shiatsu for Lovers, of course, when the participants are aware of the fingernail issue (and in any case are not performing a therapeutic massage), there are many ways to derive pleasure from long nails, and even from light scratches...

Intensive pressure on contracted areas: Sometimes, during massage, we come across areas that are very tight. Sometimes this tightness stems from incorrect posture, from prolonged sitting, from the nature of the person's work, from carrying heavy loads and lifting them incorrectly, and so on. Many practitioners want to "penetrate" these areas with a finger or palm in order to "break up" the tightness and the tension. However, these very cases should be treated in the opposite way: slowly and gently. When an area is very tight, it is naturally liable to be sensitive and sore. Invasive pressure, especially with a finger, will have the opposite effect, and the area will contract even more. This has many negative effects. The tightness makes it harder for the practitioner to release the area, the patient gets a physical "fright," his calmness and relaxation are impaired, and other areas are liable to contract again. Besides the ineffectiveness of the action, the patient suffers anguish and discomfort. Sometimes, it seems to the practitioner that as a result of the application of force to the tight, "seized up" area, he has succeeded in "releasing" it. This is not the case. Even if it looks as if the place has been released after an invasive action, it is liable to contract and revert to its previous state in a matter of seconds.

The correct way is to apply very gentle, constant, light, steady pressure to the contracted area, and penetrate it very lightly and steadily. This is especially important in Shiatsu for lovers. Working in this way is likely to take much more time, but by adopting this method, the chances of releasing the contracted area are far greater - and the patient's serenity and relaxation are not impaired.

Pressure on bones and vertebrae: Quite naturally, the patient's body will manifest a great deal of resistance, and justifiably. *We do not apply direct pressure to vertebrae, ribs, or bones.* The Shiatsu massage is performed between them only, on the soft tissues and on the muscles in a gentle and conscious way. When pressure is applied to bones, ribs, or vertebrae, the patient's body - and the patient himself - will express conscious resistance.

"Squeezing" that is too strong: One of the techniques that is used in massage is squeezing, which will be discussed at greater length later on. Sometimes, the squeezing action is too strong, hurting the patient. Again, it is important to listen to the patient's body, and to ensure that this movement does not hurt him. The squeezing does not have to be too deep. It should be very light, "catching" a quantity of tissues that are not too deep, without applying too much force. In order to increase the effectiveness of the technique and decrease the discomfort that is liable to occur, the practitioner should perform the squeezing action with a small quantity of massage oil. Using too much oil actually impairs the application of the technique, since the skin is liable to be too slippery under the practitioner's fingers, and it is not pleasant for the patient, either.

The patient's fear of touch: There are many patients whose bodies are consciously or unconsciously afraid of touch. This is common, first of all, when the patient does not know the practitioner. Second, when the patient has not had a massage or any form of touch therapy for a long time, and he needs some time to get used to his body being touched. Moreover, there are patients who, in the depths of their subconscious, have various barriers concerning touch. In Shiatsu for Lovers, this fear of touch can destroy the entire massage. In any event, when we touch the patient, and sense that he is not entirely at one with the touch, or tightens up when touched, it is important to slow the procedure down, and soothe him. This can be done by "spreading" movements (preferably using oils) - large, slow, circular movements of the entire palm on the patient's back. It is important to get him gradually accustomed to the touch of our hand.

Sometimes, it is possible to perform this kind of "preparatory massage," which includes movements such as effleurage, which we will discuss later, for quite a long time - even 20 or 30 minutes - when the patient is not used to touch or is afraid of it. If we begin to "penetrate" the soft tissues using various techniques, or use more "aggressive" techniques, the patient is liable to feel uncomfortable. The Shiatsu pressure techniques, which involve steady, slow touch with the whole palm, and concentrate on one point for seven to ten seconds, are also likely to make it easier for the patient to become familiar with our touch, as partners or practitioners, and to calm down and relax.

Modesty about exposing the body: Quite naturally, when it comes to a full body massage, there are many patients who do not feel comfortable when they have to expose their bodies. (This topic is very important in Shiatsu for Lovers.) For that reason, things should be made easier for them in every way. There could be a screen behind which they can undress, as well as suitable robes that can be put on. If there is no screen, we should leave the room while the patient is undressing, and leave a towel for him, so that he can lie down on the bed or treatment couch with the lower part of his body, or his whole body, covered. We lift the towel in order to expose the part that is to be worked on, in turn. (Female patients who do not feel comfortable about removing their bra or panties can leave their underwear on, or wear short pants, and open their bra only when their back is massaged. Male patients can keep their underwear or light, loose boxer shorts on. When a female patient turns over onto her back in order to have her chest and abdomen massaged, a narrow towel can be placed on her breasts so that she does not feel uncomfortable.) In a sexually oriented massage, in order to make the massage more pleasurable, to facilitate the feeling of enjoyment and the release of the partner who is being massaged, and also to prolong the massage procedure in order to heighten the pleasure, it is possible to start off by covering the intimate areas, and uncover them at the "right" and most appropriate time.

Oils: When we perform a massage with massage oils, we must pay attention to several things. It is very important to check that the oil is pleasing to the patient, and does not irritate or sting his skin, or cause it to itch, since this will impair his relaxation and his serenity, and a significant part of the treatment's effectiveness will be undermined. It is not always possible to drip the oil onto the patient's body. While this can be very enjoyable during an erotic massage, it is liable to disturb the patient during a therapeutic massage, and the unexpected sensation of a wet and oily substance is liable to "shock" his body.

We should spread oil or cream all over our hands, warm it up by rubbing our hands together, and only then spread it over the patient's body. On winter days, this is very important, and sometimes it is a good idea to heat the oil slightly before beginning the massage. When using massage cream, spreading it directly without warming it between the palms of the hands beforehand is liable to cause a feeling of unexpected and unpleasant coldness on the patient's body, since cream tends to be colder than massage oil.

Basic ethics

It is important to emphasize a fact that is totally obvious: Under no circumstances, and for absolutely no reason, is an erotic massage to be performed on a person who is not prepared for it, informed about it, and interested in it. Besides, of course, the possibility of being sued, both increasing "sexual energies" and any kind of sexual arousal during the treatment are absolutely forbidden when the aim of the massage is not erotic and has not been consented to by both parties. Unfortunately, there are sometimes unprofessional practitioners who consider massage a way of arousing the recipient sexually (it usually involves an amateur massage, which is not performed for purposes of physical therapy, but rather for calming and relaxing). This is reprehensible from a professional, moral, and human point of view.

Massage must not be used for performing any physical or emotional manipulations. The aim of the massage is to give, and not to "take," and there must be absolute clarity about the person's wishes and expectations concerning the massage he is about to receive. A person who performs a massage on another person without prior agreement that the aim of the massage is to arouse each other sexually, and finds *himself* sexually aroused because of his contact with the naked body, or the sight of the naked body, is obliged to stop the massage immediately. This is because he is not helping, healing or curing, but causing harm. Ultimately, this will lead to friction between him and the recipient, and a breach of trust; from the energetic point of view, there will be some kind of response that will harm the performer of the immoral massage.

Remember that the description of the massage using the Shiatsu for Lovers method that appears later on is not suitable for the first date, but rather for couples who know what to expect from each other, and do it for mutual pleasure, with full, conscious consent.

Shiatsu is performed either as a self-treatment (when the practitioner and the recipient are the same person), or as amateur Shiatsu in which there is a giver and a recipient, a practitioner and a recipient, or as professional Shiatsu, in which there is a *professional* practitioner and a recipient. In Shiatsu for Lovers, the giver is always defined as the practitioner, and the receiver as the recipient (and when they switch roles, the definitions are also switched).

Pressure methods
and massage techniques

In Shiatsu for Lovers, we will use a selection of methods that we will choose from among the pressures (four), ways of pressing (four), and massage techniques (17) that are described in the book.

The full elaboration of the methods is important - even though we do not have to use all of them - for two reasons: First, the reader will be able to choose what he most wants. Second, during the Shiatsu for Lovers massage, there are often lapses into therapeutic Shiatsu, in which a far greater variety of methods are used.

Pressure methods

1. Vertical pressure:

This is pressure applied by the practitioner to the patient, and promotes good health. It is performed by pressing the finger or the hand on the patient's body, and applying direct, vertical pressure. The advantage of this pressure is its safety. While non-vertical pressure, on the other hand, promotes the flow of blood in the body, in certain cases, there is the fear that it will impair the body's natural healing powers, especially in cases in which the patient suffers from some disease. Vertical pressure is very widespread because of its safety and its beneficial action in promoting the general health of the body.

2. Stationary pressure:

This pressure is used frequently in the Shiatsu pressure techniques. There is no movement in this pressure, and when it penetrates the body, it stimulates the parasympathetic nervous system - the system that is responsible for the conditions of calmness and relaxation. By means of this action, it soothes the nervous system and the inner organs, thus ensuring the natural flow of energy and life force in the body, and the body gains the welcome direction it needs in order to heal and balance itself.

In general, the practitioner lingers on every point for between two and seven seconds. (The length of time is measured *after* locating the point and starting to apply steady pressure to it.) This is the accepted time-length, but there are cases in which eight to thirty seconds on a point are necessary.

3. Equal pressure:

Equal pressure is created by an equal distribution of the weight and the pressure on both of the practitioner's hands. It must be remembered that the pressure does not derive from the practitioner's palms. (If we try to push with our hands only, we will soon feel pain or abrasion in these regions, especially in a Shiatsu massage.) It is important that the pressure come from the pelvis or abdomen, so that it will be steady and sure, and will not exhaust the practitioner.

When both hands are placed on the patient's body, the equal pressure principle means that while one hand is working, the other serves as a support for the practitioner's body. In this way, we transfer the weight of our body equally to both hands - 50 percent to the supporting hand, and 50 percent to the working hand. Equal pressure communicates a feeling of confidence, balance, and equilibrium to the patient, and helps him relax and calm down in the best possible way, as well as "open up" more to the pressure applied to his body by the practitioner.

4. Supporting pressure:

Supporting pressure derives from the feeling of support experienced by the practitioner himself, physically, as a result of his physical build, which attains its natural equilibrium as a result of the contraction and relaxation of his muscles. When the *practitioner* is in a state of supporting balance, while he is standing, sitting, or moving, he communicates this feeling to the patient.

The surface upon which the patient is lying or leaning also constitutes supporting pressure. (The surface has to be adapted to the purposes and manner of the treatment. Lying on a thin mattress on the floor, for example, provides a different kind of supporting pressure).

These four pressure methods constitute a basic part of the principles of Shiatsu. Since we are dealing with the combination of techniques for creating Shiatsu for Lovers - a massage combined with effective, and enjoyable pressures - we will also use the fundamental massage movements that are described in the following pages.

Massage techniques

1. Effleurage

Effleurage movements are slow, rhythmic movements, kind of light brush-strokes. To perform these movements, we mostly use the inner surface of the hand.

This movement is very suitable for the initial touch, and it can be done very softly, or much more closely to the body, so that the sliding is stronger and felt more. When effleurage is performed at the beginning of the massage, we should start with light movements. When using massage oils, effleurage is suitable for the initial spreading of the oil. By means of effleurage, it is possible to perform movements that encompass the body, and provide a feeling of warmth, protection, and tranquillity. It can be used on the back, and on the arms; both hands can be used, on each side of the patient's arm, sliding them, and applying the amount of pressure we deem appropriate. The legs can be treated in the same way. On the back and chest, large, encompassing movements should be used. It is important to remember to maintain the same pressure throughout the movement, when it is applied to a large surface, like the back. Performing this movement on the sides of the back gives the patient a wonderful feeling, especially in Shiatsu for Lovers, as if he is being "gathered" between the palms.

It is also important to remember that the fingers should not be too spread out, in order not to lose energy and power while performing the movement. In effleurage, the greater the pressure, the more effect it has on the muscles and the blood vessels. The weaker the pressure, the greater the effect on the nerves (and the less the effect on the muscles and blood vessels). Some masseurs are in the habit of beginning and ending the massage with a few effleurage movements, so as to create a warm and pleasant feeling of closing the circle, and preserving the results that were achieved during the massage.

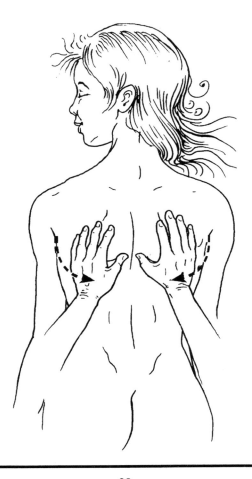

2. Kneading:

The kneading movements are reminiscent of kneading bread. They are performed by means of the whole palm and the fingers, grasping the correct amount of tissues with the hand and fingers, so as not to create a feeling of pinching. As opposed to effleurage, it is a very vigorous movement. Of course, it can be performed gently, or with greater pressure.

Too much oil spread on the area is liable to impair the movement. It releases the tissues, invigorates the blood, and works well with the muscles.

The kneading movement is performed very gently, mainly on the surface of the abdomen, and on the buttocks, the arms and the legs (on the back, a variation of this movement, called "squeezing," or petrissage, is performed), pulling the thumb in an inward direction, and the rest of the fingers, using the whole palm, in an outward direction. This is one of the most pleasant and releasing movements for the shoulders, in order to release contractions and pains.

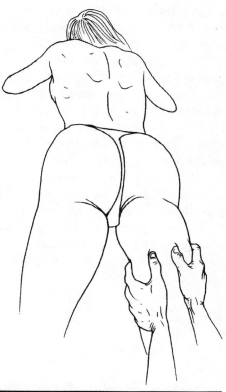

3. Squeezing (petrissage):

The petrissage movement, like effleurage, is also one of the basic movements - especially in Swedish massage and deep tissue massage. This is a most effective movement for releasing tensions and pressures in the tissues, nerves, and muscles, but a certain amount of practice is required in order to perform it in the optimal way. To perform the movement, we gently grasp the skin between the thumb and the rest of the fingers. It is better to begin it from the top and go downward, and after gaining experience and a good and correct feeling in the hands, it is possible to change the directions, using different variations, and combining petrissage with other massage techniques.

After grasping the skin between the thumb and the fingers, we squeeze it gently and let it go, using a light revolving movement beneath the fingers. This is a marvelous movement to perform on the back, and initially, it is a good idea to perform it mainly in that area, until the feeling in the hands improves. After a little experience, it can be performed on the upper part of the arm as well, and behind the thighs and the calves. (Not everyone can tolerate this movement on these areas of the body.) We must pay attention to how the patient feels about this movement.

It is important for this movement to be smooth; it begins at a particular point, and continues downward or upward along the whole surface, which produces a very effective result of loosening.

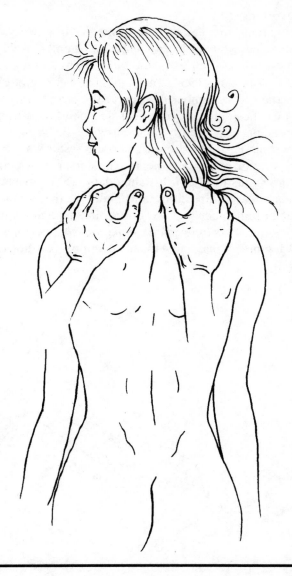

4. Revolving:

The revolving movement is used mainly in physiotherapy. It is a movement by means of which we gently, freely, and smoothly turn the joints of the body. This movement is performed on the shoulders, knees, ankles, neck, and elbows. It is important to remember to support the joint firmly. When we feel that the region is very stiff and painful, we perform the movement very gently and slowly. To complete the release, we can perform it in a lighter and faster way. By way of demonstration, think of the movements performed by a person who wants to loosen his shoulders; he revolves them a few times in one direction, and then in the other. It is important to remember that we do not massage an injured or diseased joint. *This movement must not be performed by force!* "Beginner" masseurs must be doubly cautious when applying it.

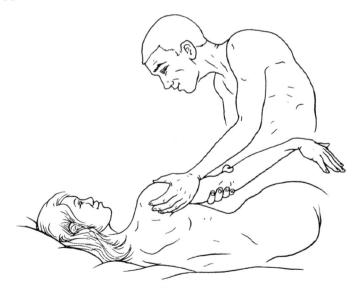

5. Rolling:

The rolling movement is a soft and releasing movement, which is applied on a relatively large surface of the body. The rolling is performed using the whole palm and all the fingers. Its aim is to move and rock relatively large areas simultaneously, and it gives a pleasant movement of relaxing the tissues and loosening them. The rolling movement is very suitable for treating the thighs, from the top down, on the back part of the calves (which are sometimes too stiff and caught to have petrissage performed on them), on the upper part of the arms, and on the buttocks. Since we can perform this movement very softly, and regulate its intensity, we should use it in order to work on areas that are too stiff to be treated by stronger movements, such as petrissage, or to "prepare the groundwork" for massage, preferably after performing a few circular and enveloping effleurage movements.

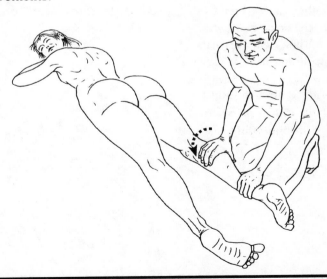

6. Rubbing-Pulling:

The rubbing-pulling movement can be used at the beginning of the massage, for preparing the body, using long, slow movements, or during the massage, for invigorating the blood (in more dynamic movements). With rubbing-pulling movements, we pass one hand, or both, over the body in a rubbing movement, while applying a little pressure. In general, the movements are performed vertically, but they can also be performed horizontally (at the sides of the back, for instance, while standing at the side of the patient). The slower and "rounder" the movement, the more relaxation and tranquillity it will provide. The faster and more vigorous it is, resembling actual rubbing, the more effective it will be in invigorating the blood. It is accepted practice to perform the movement on the back, on the sides of the back, and on the ribs (since it is not a deep movement, it can be applied to the ribs, as it does not hurt, but stimulates or soothes, according to the speed of the movement), on the chest, the arms, and the legs. When we perform the movement on the arms or legs, we can pull and rub with one hand, and hold onto the leg or hand with the other for support.

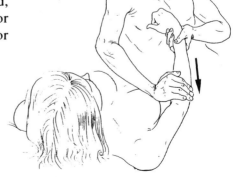

7. Turning-rubbing:

This is one of the most pleasant and soothing movements in massage. To perform the turning-rubbing we mainly use the pads of our fingers, although skilled masseurs are likely to discover that they can perform this movement on larger surfaces using the pad of the palm as well. We use the soft parts of the hand - the pads of the hands and the pads of the fingers. This movement can thus be applied to parts of the face, to the temples (using the fingers - marvelous!), with small, revolving movements on parts of the head - while sliding into the shampooing movement that will be described later, on the neck, the elbows, the knees, and the ankles. By paying a lot of attention when performing these movements, and by focusing on the fingertips that move in circular movements, both the practitioner and the patient simultaneously are likely to experience a wonderful sensation.

There is some importance to the direction of the turn, whether clockwise or anti-clockwise, and a practitioner who feels an intuitive "need" to apply the movement to a particular area in a particular direction should heed his inner feelings and act accordingly. These movements have a unique effect on the mind, especially when the massage is gentle and considerate.

8. Pulling pressure:

The pulling pressure movement is also familiar to people who practice Shiatsu. In this movement, we place both palms on the patient's back. We should start from the center of the back, when we place both palms horizontally (across the width of the patient's back, near each other), with the inner part of the palm, the hollow, over the vertebra region, so that no pressure is exerted on them. We should stand at the patient's side while performing the movement. In a vigorous and steady manner, we pull each palm in the opposite direction - one upward, all the way toward the shoulders, and the other downward, in the direction of the curve of the buttocks. The pulling movement must be clear-cut and steady, but not painful, out of sensitivity to the patient's body.

We can also perform the movement from the upper part of the thighs (where they begin) to the tip of the toes, but here we perform the pulling in a downward direction only.

Both hands can be placed gently on either side of the inner part of the knee (the hollow; not right on it, since it is a delicate area), with one hand pulling in the direction of the calf, and the other in the direction of the thigh, in a stretching movement, while they slide over those parts. This movement creates a feeling of stretching the skin and the tissues, and is likely to be very effective in relieving pain, especially after protracted physical activity.

We also use pulling pressure movements when massaging the face. Here we perform them delicately, steadily, and slowly with the *fingers*, on both sides of the patient's forehead, pulling toward the sides of the head; using almost the full length of the forefinger on each side of the bridge of the nose, pulling gently in the direction of the cheeks; and using the pads of the fingers on the eyebrows, pulling in the direction of the temples. When massaging the face, the movements are performed gently and slowly.

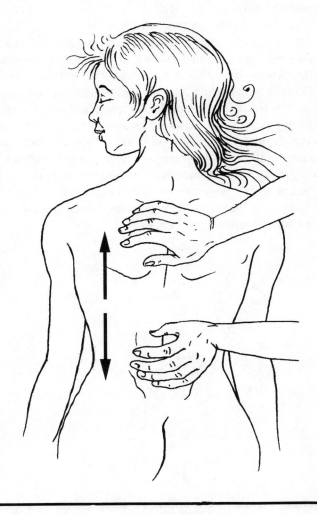

9. Shaking

Shaking movements are movements that are performed in a steady and dynamic way using both hands. They are fast movements, which can be performed on the upper part of the back, on the thighs, and on the buttocks. They are very pleasant, releasing, and dynamic. In a therapeutic massage, we try to perform the movements in the area of the buttocks and the thighs inward, in order to prevent any possible unpleasant feeling on the part of the patient in these sensitive areas. In contrast, in a sexually arousing and erotic massage, movements that are performed in an *outward* direction are likely to arouse the person sexually because they have a stimulating effect on the nerves in the thigh, buttock, and groin regions. In a therapeutic massage, we perform these movements very dynamically and at a high speed. In an erotic massage, they can be performed more slowly, so that they can work more on the nerves.

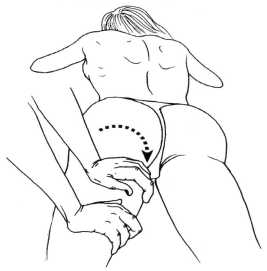

10. Tapping with the fingers:

In the tapping movements, the fingertips tap and drum on the body quickly, one after the other. This is a percussive movement, and the fingers must be spread like a rake in order to perform it and "drum" gently on the body. This movement greatly stimulates the nerve endings and invigorates the blood flow. It is performed on the whole posterior side of the body, also concentrating on the area between the shoulder joint and the chest (the area below the clavicle, in the direction of the shoulder). These movements can be performed extremely gently (only on a healthy person) on the chest region as well, in order to stimulate the thymus gland and ease congestion, and to release nervous and muscle tension in the chest. Remember that in this region, the tapping movements must be performed extremely gently and with great care.

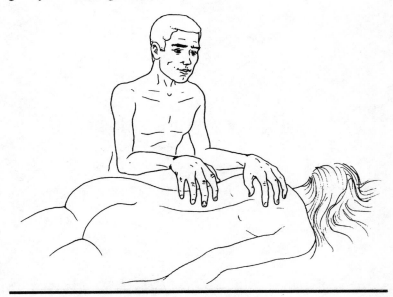

11. Tapping with cupped hands:

In this movement, we "drum" on the whole posterior side of the patient's body, so as to loosen and relax the muscles. In order to perform the movement, we curve our hands and drum with them, one at a time, creating a hollow sound.

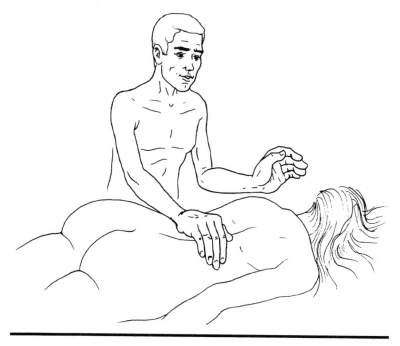

12. Slapping movement:

The slapping movements are performed on the posterior side of the patient's body quickly and alternately. To perform the movements, we flatten our hands, just like when giving a slap, but of course, we perform the movement softly, albeit with determination. These movements invigorate the blood capillaries near the surface of the skin, and the nerves that are located in the topmost layer of the skin, and cause an increase in the sensations of the skin.

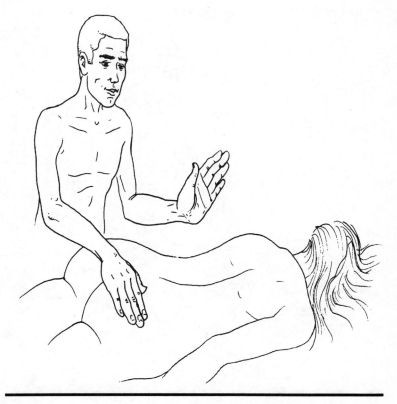

13. Chopping:

We use the chopping movement on the outer side of the hands (from the outer side of the pinkie to the outer side of the pad of the palm). These dynamic and fast movements are similar in form to karate chops, but are gentler, of course. One hand at a time, we drum on the posterior side of the patient's body, along its entire length. The movements accelerate the blood flow, and are wonderful for the circulation. After a few minutes of "drumming" using these fast movements, the patient will feel warmth and vigor, as well as tranquillity and relaxed muscles.

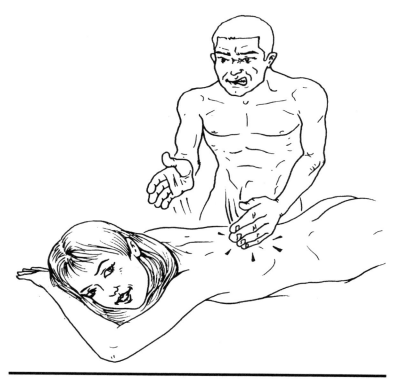

14. Pulling the nape and hair:

Despite its somewhat off-putting name, this movement does not really involve actual hair-pulling. It is a combination of two movements that create one of the most releasing movements that exist for the neck and head. To perform this movement, we stand behind the patient, who is sitting or lying on his back with his head protruding slightly from the bed, and we gently grasp his nape with two hands. We gently pull one hand at a time, sliding them upward along the nape, moving them in a bold movement along the back of the head, and lightly pulling the roots of the hair (a gentle pull, while grasping the hair as near as possible to the roots), and ending the movement by passing the fingers through the hair, separating the strands and pulling them lightly and gently. When this movement is performed well, and we listen really attentively to the patient's body and to the movements of our own hands, it is a wonderful release for the head and neck.

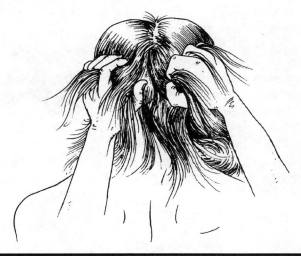

15. Shampooing:

The shampooing movement, which is performed on the scalp, is familiar to many people from the beauty salon or the barber shop. Of course, during massage, we do not perform these movements quickly or perfunctorily, but slowly, with a good instinct for the stiff areas of the patient's scalp. To perform the movement, we have to stand, or sit (more comfortable from the point of view of height) behind the patient's head, when he is lying on his back with his head protruding slightly from the bed. The movement is performed using the fingers and the pads of the hands. We gently ease our fingers between the patient's strands of hair, preferably starting from the bottom - from the place where the head joins the neck, and we begin to rib and massage the delicate tissue of the scalp with soft, circular movements. A little bit of pressure can be applied, but we must remember to support the patient's head with the pads of our palms, while the fingers perform the shampooing movement. It is possible to perform vigorous movements that stimulate, invigorate, and increase alertness.

Soft, slow, rhythmical movements induce a state of deep relaxation (in certain cases, a state of alpha waves). Some people use this movement before a guided visualization, for example, because of the deep relaxation it induces.

It is a wonderful way of releasing the many tensions that concentrate in the region of the head.

16. Neuromuscular massage on both sides of the spinal column:

This massage aims to release the muscles, the tendons, the connective tissue, and the nerves. It is performed mainly by the fingers, but also by the pads of the hands, and it must be performed extremely carefully. When the practitioner is experienced, he can also find the specific points along the spinal column that are stiff. We begin from the top of the spinal column - *under no circumstances along the spinal column itself, but on each side.* At the beginning of the massage, when using the fingers, and the body is not yet relaxed and loose enough, the movements must be performed with the fingers with extreme gentleness; pressure can be used, but it must be gentle pressure that is not too invasive, because we will probably encounter many stiff points on our way, and penetrating them too deeply with our fingers is liable to hurt the patient.

After we have performed this technique several times, or feel that the muscles on both sides of the spinal column are looser, we can use our fingers to penetrate a bit into the places where we felt some kind of stiffness. The penetration is performed by placing the pad of the finger on the point, and applying a steady, slow pressure inward for a number of seconds.

In the same slow manner in which we entered the tissue, we also leave it.

To perform this technique, a great deal of sensitivity in the hands is required, as well as an ability to feel the patient's body in the correct way. Beginner masseurs must first perform the movements with extreme gentleness, more in order to learn than to loosen muscles, until they learn how to perform this technique correctly without hurting the patient.

By using this technique, we can release muscles, connective tissues, and nerves very successfully. We must remember that when we press on a nerve, we affect all the organs and areas it serves. An inexperienced masseur - especially an amateur - must not begin with deep, penetrative finger work. He can simply pull his fingers slowly along the spinal column in order to release the connective tissue, the muscles, and the nerves that are nearer the surface.

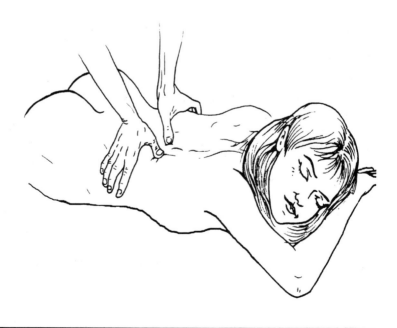

17. Feathering:

Feathering movements are used mainly during a sexually arousing massage, and can be used at various stages of Shiatsu for Lovers - at the beginning or end of a process, or in combination with other pressures.

This technique is especially pleasurable, as it stimulates the nerve endings and soothes the body. However, there are people who cannot tolerate it because of the extreme sensitivity of their nerves. It is therefore important to pay attention to the reaction of one's patient or partner (in an erotic massage) when performing the movement.

To perform this movement, we use a long feather (such as an ostrich feather), a silk scarf, a piece of fur, or a soft, thick brush. In fact, it is possible to experiment with a range of soft, pleasant brushes. We move the object along our partner's entire body, creating a pleasurable, slightly ticklish sensation. The movement can also be performed with the fingertips, in a fluttering motion, concentrating on the erogenous zones. It is highly recommended in Shiatsu for Lovers. (A tip for "professionals": Use your tongue, hair, eyelashes, pubic hair, nipples, or penis for feathering.)

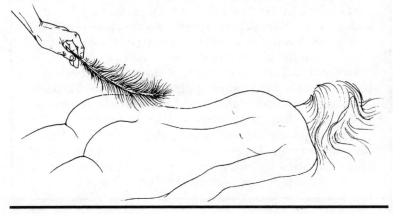

Essential points

General Shiatsu massage is the starting point for Shiatsu for Lovers. After the general massage, and sometimes unrelated to it, we move on to specific massage - both for increasing the effect in particular fields that suit the purpose of the massage, and for overcoming problems and obstacles.

In Shiatsu for Lovers, this specific massage includes massaging areas in which the essential points are located, as explained below. Specific massage in Shiatsu for Lovers can also take the form of a general feathering of the entire body, or any other massage technique - wherever your imagination takes you!

After the massage, we move on to Shiatsu for Lovers, which is based on pressures. To this end, we have to be familiar with 24 essential points in the body. These points are effective during love-making, as well as for relieving menstrual cramps and other pains and symptoms that accompany the monthly period, impotence, premature ejaculation, and so on.

Unless indicated otherwise, the points are located on both sides of the body: that is, on both legs, on both hands, and so on, in parallel locations. The exceptions are the points that are located in the center of the body: on the abdomen, the nose, and so on.
In the illustrations, only one of the pair of points is shown. You should always apply pressure to both points - for example, above the right knee and above the left knee - even though pressure applied to only one of the pair of points will also lead to the desired results.
In cases where it is specifically indicated that pressure must be applied to both points, you must ensure that you do this (point number 15, for instance).

1. The "Intersection of the Three Yins" point:

This point is effective in relieving menstrual cramps, period pains, and various emotional and physical symptoms that occur several days before - as well as during - it.

This point is located four finger-widths above the inner ankle bone, behind the tibia (the inner calf bone) on both legs. Vertical pressure is applied to this point with the thumb on the point, and the fingers serving as supports. (Some people call this the "pinching" technique, because the thumb and fingers create "pincers.") Pressure should be applied gradually, from light to medium, keeping the thumb on the point for seven seconds, and gradually releasing the pressure without detaching the thumb from the point. The procedure should be repeated several times.

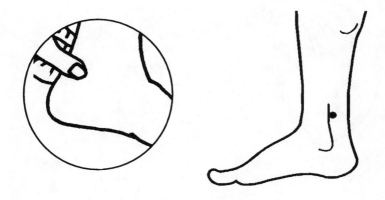

2. The "Sea of Blood" point:

This important point, which is located above the knee, on the inner side of both legs, serves to fortify women generally, and to relieve menstrual symptoms, cramps, pains, and fluctuations in their emotional state a few days before as well as during the period.

Pressure is applied to this point while the woman is seated on a chair. Her partner covers her kneecap with his hand. The point is located below his thumb, when he is sitting on the floor (or on a cushion) in front of her. Pressure is applied gradually, keeping the thumb on the point for several seconds, and gradually releasing the pressure without detaching the thumb from the point. The procedure should be repeated.

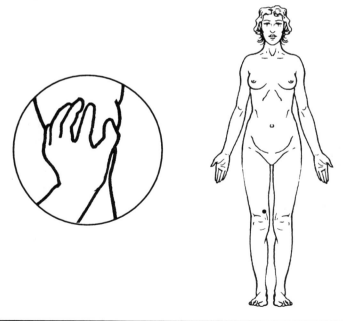

3. The "Original Chi" point*:

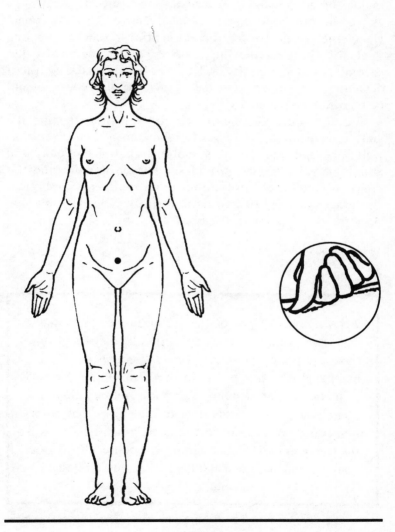

This important point, which fortifies the body in general, and has many therapeutic advantages, is located in the middle of the abdomen, at a distance of three finger-widths above the big bone that is situated above the pubic bone. Using the thumb or forefinger, gentle pressure is applied gradually, keeping the finger on the point for five to ten seconds, and gradually releasing the pressure without detaching the finger from the point. The procedure should be repeated several times.

Besides being an important point for strengthening the body in general, it also serves to relieve menstrual cramps, as well as other pains and symptoms that accompany the monthly cycle. It also provides relief during the mid-life crisis of men, by providing them with psychological encouragement and overall reinforcement. There is only one "Original Chi" point in the body.

*A number of points that are located close to one another on the abdomen are difficult to distinguish . Those are points number 3, 5, 6, 7, and they are close to number 8 (the five points of the "Conception Vessel" meridian, not including Hui Yin) - in fact, almost "touching" it. It is important to remember that points number 3, 5, 6, 7 are treated separately, while number 8 - the five points in a row - are treated consecutively, and sometimes with one application of pressure (again, excluding Hui Yin).

4. The "Walking Three Miles" point:

This point is located at a distance of four finger-widths below the kneecap (while sitting on a chair) on both legs. It is located exactly where the fourth finger encounters the tibia, that is, on the edge of the bone toward the inner part of the leg. With fingers enveloping the kneecap, gradual pressure is applied with the thumb, keeping it on the point, and gradually releasing the pressure without detaching the thumb from the point.

The procedure should be repeated several times.

This point is very important, and is also used for general strengthening, and for relieving menstrual pains and cramps as well as other symptoms that accompany the monthly cycle. It also provides relief during the mid-life crisis of men, and fortifies them generally.

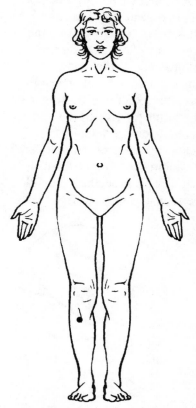

5. The "Pass Organ" point:

This important point strengthens the body in general, increases virility, improves sexual performance, and increases sexual arousal during intercourse. It is an excellent point for daily practice in order to improve general sexual functioning.

It is located in the center of the abdomen, just below the navel. Gentle pressure can be applied gradually with the thumb, the forefinger, or the top joint of the forefinger reinforced by the middle finger in order to increase the pressure, keeping the finger on the point for five to ten seconds, and gradually releasing the pressure without detaching the finger from the point. The procedure should be repeated three to five times.

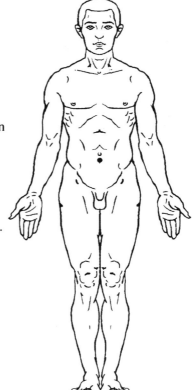

6. The "Middle Extreme" point:

In daily practice, pressure on this point helps to increase sexual vigor and to improve sexual function. When pressure is applied to it during foreplay, it is extremely arousing. The point is located in the center of the slope of the abdomen, directly above the pubic bone. There is only one "Middle Extreme" point in the body.

Gentle pressure can be applied gradually with the thumb, the forefinger, or the top joint of the forefinger reinforced by the middle finger in order to increase the pressure, keeping the finger on the point for several seconds, and gradually releasing the pressure without detaching the finger from the point. The procedure should be repeated several times.

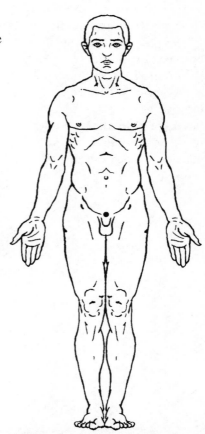

7. The "Crooked Bone" point:

This point is located at a distance of two finger-widths above the "Middle Extreme" point. Gentle pressure is applied gradually with the thumb, the forefinger, or the top joint of the forefinger reinforced by the middle finger in order to increase the pressure, keeping the finger on the point for several seconds, and gradually releasing the pressure without detaching the finger from the point.

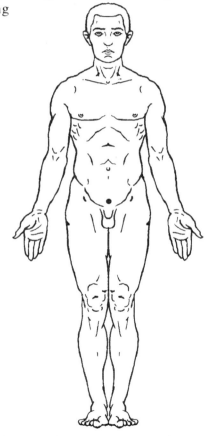

The procedure should be repeated several times.

In daily practice, pressure on this point serves to improve general sexual functioning, to enhance and fortify sexual vigor, and to increase arousal during foreplay.

8. The "Conception Vessel" point:

This point actually consists of several points, which are also known as perineal points, the most important of which is the perineal or "Conception Vessel One" point. These are the most important points in erotic stimulation and for treating various kinds of sexual problems. The "Conception Vessel" meridian is located along the central line of the lower abdomen, and along it are the five most important

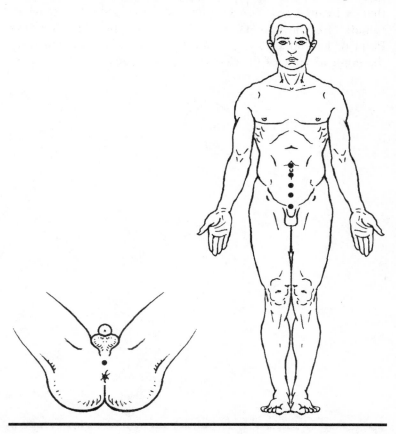

points for sexual arousal. They can be used for foreplay preceding intercourse, or for strengthening and balancing the sexual system on a daily basis. The points begin from the pubic bone, along the central line, and ascend to a distance of two finger-widths above the navel. Pressure can be applied to the points with the forefinger or the palm.

However, the point that is considered the most significant for sexual arousal during foreplay and intercourse is the one that is located between the anus and the genitals - male or female. Its Chinese name is "Hui Yin," or "The Meeting Point of Feminine Power," and it is extremely powerful from the point of view of the sexual arousal it causes.

9. The pressure point below the knee:

This pressure point is located below the knee, slightly in the direction of the inner side of the leg. It is very effective in relieving menstrual cramps, as well as other pains and symptoms that accompany the monthly period. Pressure should be applied to this point with the thumb for a few seconds. The point is located on both legs.

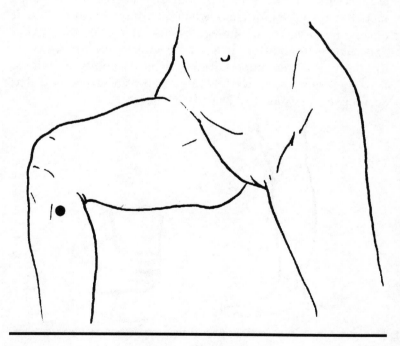

10. The pressure point at the base of the calf:

This pressure point is located at the base of the calf on both legs, on its lowest part, and on the inner side of the leg, at a distance of about four finger-widths above the ankle, close to the tibia, but not on it. It is very easy to apply "pinching" pressure to this point, but pressure can also be applied with the forefinger, or with the top joint of the forefinger reinforced by the middle finger in order to increase the pressure, keeping the finger on the point for about seven seconds, and gradually releasing the pressure without detaching the finger from the point. The procedure should be repeated several times.

If pressure is applied to this point on a daily basis, all aspects of sexual function will improve considerably. It helps increase sexual vigor, and when pressure is applied to it during intercourse, it augments and intensifies the sexual experience. In addition, it has a general fortifying effect on the body. Another important action is its ability to relieve menstrual cramps, as well as other pains and symptoms that accompany the monthly period.

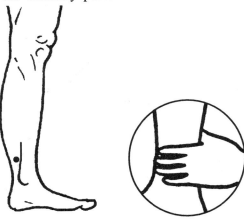

11. The pressure point on the outer side of the calf:

This pressure point is located at a distance of three finger-widths below the kneecap on both legs, in the direction of the outer side of the calf, close to the tibia, but not on it. Pressure is applied to the point in a sitting position, with the hand covering the kneecap, and the thumb applying the pressure. Pressure is applied gradually several times, keeping the thumb on the point for about five to ten seconds, gradually releasing the pressure without detaching the thumb from the point.

Daily practice on this point improves all aspects of sexual functioning, and increases sexual vigor. Pressure can be applied during intercourse, in order to augment the sexual experience. In addition, this point has an important and varied action for strengthening all the body's functions, and it is very effective for soothing and alleviating inner agitation.

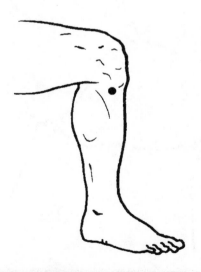

12. The pressure point above the knee:

This pressure point is located above the knee, toward the inner part of both legs. This point is also used for relieving menstrual cramps, as well as other pains and symptoms that accompany the monthly period. Pressure is applied by covering the knee with the hand, and the thumb applying gradual pressure, keeping it on the point for seven to ten seconds, and gradually releasing the pressure without detaching the thumb from the point. The procedure is repeated three to five times.

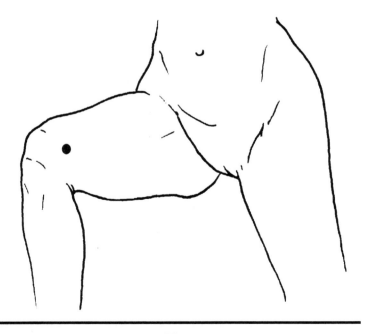

13. The pressure point on the outer side of the thigh:

This pressure point is located on the outer side of both thighs, a little in from the crease of the buttocks. This is another point which helps relieve menstrual cramps, as well as other pains and symptoms that accompany the monthly period. Sometimes it is easier to have a partner apply pressure, when the recipient is standing. Pressure can be applied to the point when the palm is placed at the base of the buttocks, spread out, and the thumb applies gradual pressure to the point, and remains there for about seven seconds. The pressure is released gradually without detaching the thumb from the point. The procedure is repeated at least three times.

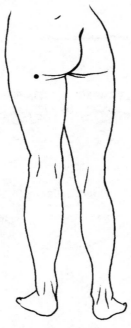

14. The pressure point at the top of the bridge of the nose:

This pressure point is located at the top of the bridge of the nose, between the eyebrows. It is used for relieving menopausal symptoms such as hot and cold flashes, backaches, tremors, sudden feelings of exhaustion, and other symptoms. In addition, it helps significantly in alleviating the emotional aspects of men's mid-life crisis. There is only one point like this in the body.

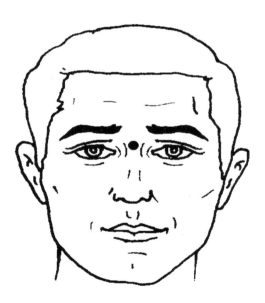

15. The pressure point on the sole of the foot:

This pressure point is located between the two pads of the sole of the foot, slightly toward the big toe on both feet. *Pressure must be applied to the points on both feet.* The point is used for alleviating menopausal symptoms - both physical and emotional.

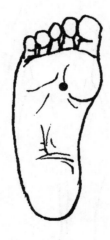

16. The stomach meridian pressure points:

One point is located next to the area of the pubic bone (pelvis), and the second below the knee. Pressure is applied to this point for sexual arousal, mainly in cases of frigidity. Despite the distance between the two points, they must both be treated together (if possible), or one after the other.

Note that on each leg, there are two stomach meridian points.

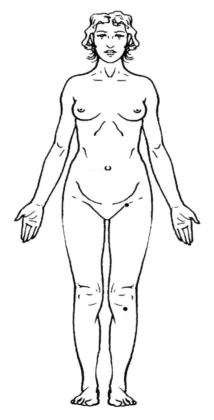

17. The liver meridian pressure point:

This pressure point is located on both thighs, slightly below the pelvis in front. (It tends slightly toward the inner part of the thigh.) It serves to increase sexual arousal and helps in cases of frigidity.

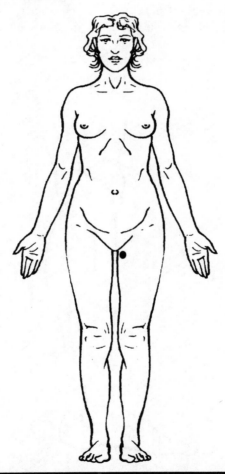

18. The spleen meridian pressure points:

A pair of points: one point is located on the inner part of the leg next to the knee, and the other on the meridian above the ankle. Both of these points help in cases of frigidity. Despite the distance between the two points, they must both be treated together (if possible), or one after the other.

Note that on each leg, there are two spleen meridian points.

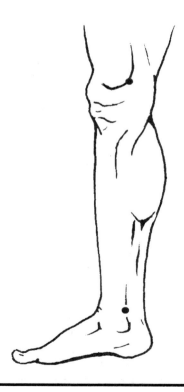

19. The pressure points on the back:

There are many pressure points located on the back, and they are connected to the nerves that supply energy to the reproductive organs. These nerves, together with the nerves in the lower back region, control almost all the vital functions of the lower region of the body, such as urination, erection,

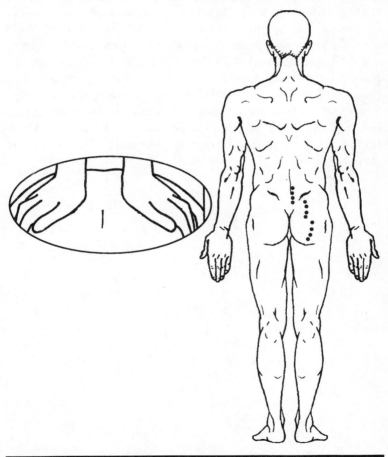

copulation, and so on. Pressure is applied with the whole palm, preferably with all the fingers simultaneously. In this way, we can treat a large number of points at the same time. Light to medium pressure should be applied, while using all the fingers to apply pressure to the following areas: both sides of the spinal column, right next to the vertebrae, from slightly below the waist down to above the end of the coccyx (a palm's length above the coccyx); at a distance of about three finger-widths from this point (when the palm is placed vertically on the area), a bit lower than the first point, again a palm's length; and a third point, at a distance of about three finger-widths (when the hand is held vertically on the body), at a point a bit lower, so that the whole spread hand almost reaches the base of the crease of the buttocks. These important points are extremely effective for increasing sexual arousal.

20. The pressure points on the upper thigh:

The pressure points on the thighs, especially at the front of the thighs, are also connected to the kidney, spleen, and other meridians. These points are numerous, and in order to stimulate most of them simultaneously, gentle pressure must be applied to the inner front area of the thighs. In order to stimulate them, it is possible to apply pressure in a variety of ways - by steady pressure, by stroking, or by massage. They are very effective in sexual arousal, and give a new flavor to foreplay. Pressure can also be applied to them during intercourse, in order to intensify the experience.

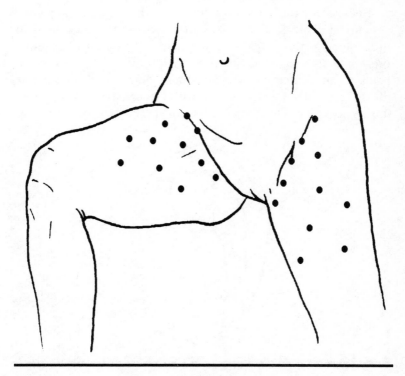

21. The pressure points on the ear:

There are numerous nerves on the surface of the outer ear, one of which is connected to the autonomic nervous system, which also plays a role in the various actions of the sexual system. (This particular point is illustrated below. The rest of the points are not indicated.)

Applying pressure to the area of the ear that is parallel to the temple is effective for treating various states of sexual inadequacy, and various problems in sexual functioning. In addition, like the rest of the points on the ear, it also helps increase sexual desire, both during foreplay and generally, when the pressure is applied on a daily basis.

Because of the numerous points in this area, it is a good idea to apply different forms of touch to the ear, such as nibbling on the ear, kissing, sucking, touching, gentle pressure, and so on. Touching the points on the outer ear leads to an increase in sexual arousal and an intensification of the sexual experience, as well as creating stimulation during foreplay. Of course, let's not forget that there are two ears!

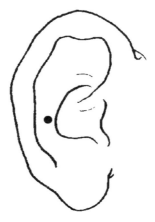

22. The pressure points on the hand:

The action of this pressure point is widespread and varied, and it reinforces all the functions of the body. It is located on the gap between the thumb and the forefinger on both hands, slightly in the direction of the root of the palm, at a distance of a finger-width below the first joint of the forefinger, on the outer part of the hand, parallel to the bone, but not on it. Pressure should be applied using the "pinching" technique, when the practitioner's forefinger is placed above the pad of the patient's thumb, and pressure is applied with the practitioner's thumb on this point. Both hands should be pressed each time, for a few seconds, and the procedure should be repeated several times without detaching the thumb from the point.

This point serves to fortify and balance the body in general, and daily practice will result in an improvement in all aspects of sexual functioning. The point is also used for increasing sexual vigor, and pressure can be applied to it during intercourse in order to intensify the sexual experience.

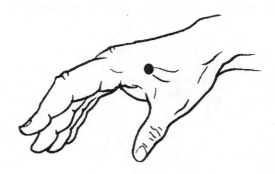

23. **The pressure point between the eyebrows:**

This point is situated exactly between the eyebrows, at the end of the bridge of the nose - not actually on it, but just above it. The bone can be felt below the pressure point. This point is very effective in reducing tension, nervousness, and pressure, and is helpful in relieving headaches. There is one point like this in the body.

Since it is very soothing, it contributes indirectly to increasing the body's vitality and to increasing sexual strength. When pressure is applied to it before intercourse or during foreplay, it increases the enjoyment and the ability to shake off everyday cares, and to concentrate on sexual pleasure. Because of these soothing properties, it is also helpful in cases of loss of libido or a drop in sexual pleasure as a result of tension or anxiety.

Pressure can be applied to this point with the thumb, but it is easier to use the forefinger or the middle finger. It is also possible to apply pressure with the top joint of the forefinger reinforced by the middle finger to increase the pressure. Gradual pressure should be applied to the point, keeping the finger on the point for a few seconds, and gradually releasing the pressure without detaching the finger from the point. The procedure should be repeated several times.

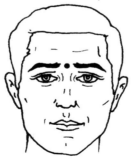

24. The pressure point between the upper lip and the nose:

This point is situated in the indentation between the upper lip and the nose. It helps considerably in releasing tensions and pressures, and in attaining a state of calmness and serenity. In addition, it is known as a point that contributes to the stimulation of facial beauty and the skin of the face. There is one point like this in the body.

Gradual, gentle pressure should be applied to this point, and the pressure should be released gradually without detaching the finger from the point. The procedure should be repeated several times.

By means of its soothing action, this point helps increase sexual power, enjoyment during intercourse, and the ability to concentrate on sexual pleasure. Moreover, it helps increase the body's vitality. It is recommended for use in various problems of a decrease in libido and sexual arousal, which are linked to the psychological aspects of anxiety and tension.

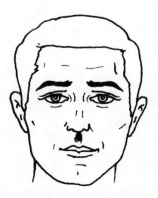

These 24 points are the central points in Shiatsu for Lovers. In the second part of the book, which is devoted only to Shiatsu for Lovers, we will emphasize some of these points (for the purpose of specific treatment), and elaborate upon the massage and its effects - at the risk of some repetition.

Note that some of the points are close to each other - for example, number 23 is close to and above number 14; numbers 1-10 are very close together, and so on. As a result, when we apply pressure to one point, we sometimes activate the point that is close to it. This is not in the least harmful.

A massage using oils and essential oils

Oils and essential oils have marvelous effects on the mind and body. Every massage performed with oils is likely to be more effective than a massage without them, because it combines the advantages of the massage itself, as well as the properties of the oils. Massage is also a widespread and accepted way of getting the oils to penetrate the body via the skin. Massage combines touch, which in itself is a therapeutic aspect - both physical and mental - with the action of the oils. In the case of various pains, especially muscle pains, the relief that is brought about by massage with essential oils is more significant, as are conditions that necessitate the reduction of swelling and congestion. Massage causes a sensation of general calmness and relaxation, and, in accordance with the choice of oils, is even likely to help the person feel more alert and energetic. On the mental plane, massage helps remove energetic blockages, reduce mental tension, release mental reactions, and raise the energetic-vital level.

When we treat sexual problems, the combination of massage with Shiatsu pressure points, and with the correct mixture of essential oils, is likely to lead to a more rapid, effective, and comprehensive result. There are many types of essential oils that we can use in massage in order to attain a good feeling of calmness that will facilitate the solution of sexual problems; we can also use essential oils with aphrodisiac properties.

Essential oils are very important in Shiatsu for Lovers. Certain oils have aphrodisiac properties, that is, they are sexual stimulants that are very powerful, especially during a Shiatsu massage whose aim is to bring about sexual arousal.

When we combine essential oils with a massage, we must remember several important rules.

Essential oils have different levels of toxicity, and no oil must be spread directly on the body.

Because of the toxicity of the oils, we only use them when they have been mixed with vegetable oils.

There is a large variety of vegetable oils, which have their own beneficial and healing properties. In addition, during massage with oils, vegetable oils are also important for significantly facilitating the massage action. The hand slides more easily, the sensation is warmer and more pleasant, and the effect is different - possible even nicer - than during a massage without oils. Moreover, the use of oils during massage is simpler, more pleasant, and more convenient than the use of various creams.

There are numerous different types of vegetable oils, and when we prepare a mixture for massage, which also contains essential oils, we take into account the properties of the vegetable oils in order to receive a better and more effective result.

In general, a higher percentage of the vegetable oil mixture is a vegetable oil with a greater absorption capacity, so that massaging the oils into the skin is easier and more effective. Moreover, we have to be aware of the odor of the vegetable oil; if it has a pungent odor, we do not use it for facial treatments, and sometimes not even for general massage - or we only use the smallest amount.

Following is a variety of vegetable oils that constitute a good basis for preparing a mixture for massage. They can also be used without the addition of essential oils, in order to facilitate the massage action (but when they are combined with essential oils, the results are wonderful).

❏ **Sweet almond oil** is absorbed well in the body, has a pleasant texture, is almost odorless, and is suitable for a general body massage.

❏ **Grape seed oil** is absorbed well in the body, has a pleasant texture, is almost odorless, and is suitable for a general body massage.

❏ **Apricot kernel oil** is absorbed well in the body, has a very delicate and pleasant texture, and is almost odorless.

❏ **Peach kernel oil** is absorbed well in the body, has a very delicate and pleasant texture, and is almost odorless.

❏ **Sesame oil** has a very high mineral and vitamin content, but because of its density and its relatively low absorption capacity in the body, it is used only as an additive to a mixture of **vegetable** oils.

❏ **Avocado oil** has a relatively high vitamin and mineral content, but its absorption capacity is low.

❏ **Wheat-germ oil**, which is rich in minerals and vitamins, has important healing properties for the body and the skin, and also serves as an antioxidant and a preservative for mixtures of oils that are kept in little bottles. However, it is dense and thick, and its absorption capacity in the body is low, so it constitutes no more than 20% of the overall mixture.

❐ **Olive oil** is used only in rare instances when the person is suffering from a severe pain somewhere in his body. It has unique healing properties, but it is very thick, is not easily absorbed in the body, and has a dominant odor.

It is worth mentioning the cosmetic oils, of which we add a few drops or small quantities to the general mixture of vegetable oils or vegetable oils and essential oils, in order to add the effect of beauty and elasticity, as well as the healing of sores and a certain degree of smoothing out wrinkles, during massage for treating the skin. The following essential oils belong to this group:

❐ **Evening Primrose oil**
❐ **Rose-hip oil**
❐ **Passionflower oil**
❐ **Gold of Pleasure oil**
❐ **Borage oil**
❐ **Cherry kernel oil.**

After choosing a suitable vegetable oil for the massage we wish to perform, we choose a number of appropriate essential oils. To prepare the mixture, we use no more than four essential oils at a time, diluted with the vegetable oil. It is possible, of course, to use only one essential oil, but a combination of up to four of them in the mixture enables us to strengthen the mixture and balance it, to treat different aspects of the massage at the same time - such as soothing, sexual arousal, muscle pains, and so on.

When we prepare a mixture from several essential oils, we must ensure that the oils are suitable for the general purpose of the massage, such as soothing, sexual arousal, and so on.

No less important is to ensure that the mixture is balanced in its odor and strength.

To prepare the mixture itself, we always use a double quantity of cc (ml) of vegetable oil to one drop of essential oil. For example, for four drops of essential oil (or one drop each of four essential oils), we use 8 cc of vegetable oil or mixture of vegetable oils.

Before we describe the sexually arousing oils, here is a brief list of oils that do other important things that can be useful to us during massage.

First of all, we will mention the *soothing oils*: grapefruit, bergamot, lavender, ylang-ylang (a wonderful oil that is also a delicate sexual stimulant), benzoin, angelica, Syberian fir, lemon, marjoram, melissa, mandarin, nerouli (bitter orange), cedarwood, sandalwood, petitgrain, patchouli (also counted as a sexually stimulating oil, but not everyone is fond of its odor), clary sage, chamomile, orange, rosewood, frankincense, lemon grass, parsley, jasmine, louisa, myrrh, bay leaves, rose, rosewater, vetiver, and tangerine. In general, all citrus oils have a soothing effect on both mind and body.

An additional type of oils that is used during massage is the group of *invigorating oils*. During a sexually arousing massage, we can combine them in a mixture that contains soothing and aphrodisiac oils, so that at the end of the massage, the person will not be too sleepy to continue enjoying himself. The invigorating essential oils include: peppermint (when used in small quantities), cajeput, patchouli (which is both soothing and sexually arousing in a gentle way), petitgrain, eucalyptus, cedarwood, grapefruit (which is also soothing), bergamot (which is also soothing), wintergreen, ginger, everlasting, galbanum, coriander, frankincense (which is also soothing), lemon (both soothing and invigorating), mandarin, marigold (which is also soothing), niaouli, mint, juniper, black pepper, citronella, clove, red thyme, caraway, cinnamon, camphor, cardamom, and rosemary.

When one of the aims of the massage is to relieve pains in the muscles or limbs, we add one of the *anesthetic oils* to the mixture, since these help reduce and relieve the pain. The following are anesthetic oils: galbanum, lavender (which also helps with the general fortifying of the body, as well as calming the body and mind), birch, niaouli, celery, bay, delicate and pleasant chamomile, rosewood with its marvelous cosmetic properties, and stimulating rosemary.

Sexually arousing oils

Throughout history, sexually arousing oils have been used. They were considered the "secret weapon" of the famous seductresses, who were in the habit of anointing their bodies and their lovers' bodies with them in order to intensify the seduction, the arousal, and the sexual passion, and to render themselves irresistible. Moreover, besides the wonderful effect that these oils have on people who do not suffer from any libido problems or lack of sexual arousal, the use of sexually arousing oils can help treat people who are experiencing a drop in their libido or any other problems in this area.

Problems of a lack of libido - whether generally, before intercourse, or during intercourse - are complex phenomena, which are liable to be caused by an extremely broad range of factors, some physiological and some psychological (significantly more frequently). Cases in which the situation is not critical in the least are very common, such as couples who feel "bored" and experience a drop in their libido, after having had sexual relations over a long period of time.

Sometimes, a lack of libido is liable to stem from daily worries, agitation, difficulty in winding down and forgetting everything, and simply concentrating on enjoyable sensations.

When it is a matter of physical problems (such as vaginismus, vaginal burning, pains during intercourse that cause a fear of sex, and so on) or psychological ones (and these are many, ranging from sexual traumas or a feeling of guilt during sex, to a fear of losing control, and so on), it is important to identify them and seek the appropriate holistic, medical, or psychological help.

The contribution of essential oils to increasing libido is exceptionally successful. Besides the calmness that treats one group of significant problems that impair enjoyable sexual relations - tension, pressure, anxiety, inability to relax and let go, and so on - some of the essential oils have amazing properties in the field of sexual arousal. These oils are called *aphrodisiacs*, and have been used for hundreds of years. There are many stories and legends about their powers of attraction and ability to stimulate libido. Whoever tries out these oils is likely to discover that there is a great deal of truth in the stories...

Among the known aphrodisiac oils, some have a greater effect on one particular person, while others have a greater effect on another. There is a large selection of sexually arousing essential oils, and in the following list you will certainly find one or more that suit both of you.

❐ The first is rose, which is a luxurious oil, and is mainly used for the sexual arousal of the woman. It is reputed to inspire in her a feeling of warmth and of confidence in her own sexuality. (It is important to distinguish between "absolute" rose oil, which is pure, and extremely expensive, and synthetic and diluted oils, or rose water, whose effectiveness is significantly lower.)

❐ The second oil famous for its aphrodisiac properties is jasmine. This oil is used to arouse men sexually, but works the same for women. This oil is also luxurious and costly, and one must beware of imitations.

❐ Ylang ylang oil, with its wonderful fragrance, is a very effective aphrodisiac. There are women who are in the habit of sprinkling ylang ylang oil diluted in vegetable oil on their labia in order to increase their sexual arousal and pleasure significantly.

❒ Patchouli oil is also a very effective aphrodisiac, but when it comes to sprinkling it on the body, it is important to check that its odor is pleasing to both members of the couple, since there are people who adore the unusual smell, and others who cannot tolerate it.

❒ Similarly, cedarwood, vetiver, ginger, clary sage, nerouli, and sandalwood are aphrodisiac oils.

It is possible to use essential oils in a variety of ways for arousing passion and sexual desire. First of all, they are very powerful when used during massage. They are likely to arouse both the masseur and the recipient. A bath containing about eight drops of aphrodisiac essential oils, before the massage or before going to bed, alone or together, is likely to be fantastically enjoyable.

Another method of increasing libido, and of adding another enjoyable dimension to sexual activity, is by burning oil in an essential oil burner. The burner is filled with water, with a candle underneath it. Ten drops of essential oils are placed in the water in the burner, and the candle is lit. The burner gives off pleasant and sexually arousing odors in the room, and is likely to contribute greatly to the increase of pleasure and sexual desire.

Remember that massage must not be performed without diluting the oils in vegetable oil, and moreover, that condoms must not come into contact with essential oils, as the oils damage the rubber.

Who can be treated with massage (and who can't)?

Since massage is a very powerful treatment that exerts a strong influence on the body, there are cases in which it must not be used.

❐ Viral infections or inflammations at an acute stage.

❐ A high fever.

❐ Bruises, open wounds, and burns.

❐ Every heart disease, even in situations of recovery after a heart disease or surgery, and pacemakers.

❐ Transplanted organs.

❐ Shrapnel or platina in the body.

❐ Acute diseases (such as pneumonia), for which medications are taken.

❐ Patients who take "cocktails" of drugs, such as certain cases of diabetes and AIDS.

❐ Surgery on internal organs, which precludes massage for six months; consult with the patient's physician.

❐ Treatment of cancer patients; consult with the patient's physician.

❐ Inflamed, congested, and swollen areas, such as a sprain or a fracture.

❐ Highly inflamed veins, and varicose veins in a state of inflammation.

❐ Pregnant women should only be treated by practitioners who have learned specific techniques for treating pregnant women.

Preparation and method of massage

Massage is a very intimate treatment, and the patient's or partner's feeling during the treatment - that is, if the patient is calm, relaxed, and serene - is of cardinal importance to its success.

The atmosphere of the room in which the massage is being performed has a significant effect on the patient's level of calmness, and the calmer and more comfortable he is, the more effective the treatment will be. To this end, we have to ensure that the room is well aired, with a pleasant odor.

Since part of the patient's body is exposed during the massage (the part that is not being massaged must be covered with a sheet or a towel), it is important for the temperature of the room to be comfortable. Cold is liable to impair the masseur's work, as it can cause the patient to feel uncomfortable, make it difficult for him to relax, and, worst of all, cause his muscles to contract, which can severely undermine the success of the treatment. If the practitioner (the giver of the massage) is also exposed, the cold will make things difficult for him, too.

The lighting in the room must be dim, relaxing, and unobtrusive. Soothing, relaxing music can be wonderful during the treatment, and is sometimes very important for people who are slightly afraid of physical contact. In any event, it is important to agree about music, volume, and type.

It is important both for the patient and for the practitioner to perform the massage on a suitable bed, which affords convenient access to all the massage areas, and does not break the practitioner's back. (From that one, it is possible to move on to another bed.) The standard massage bed is ideal for this. When we perform an erotic and arousing massage on our partner, a double bed is also a good solution, as long as it is not so soft that we cannot sit comfortably next to our partner on it. If the bed is too soft, the balance of the partner performing the massage is liable to be impaired.

It is important to see that the bed-linen is clean and pleasant, and when essential oils are used during the massage, it is a good idea to use a disposable sheet so that the oil does not stain the bed-linen.

When we are preparing for Shiatsu for Lovers, for sexual arousal, it is very important to prepare the background for the massage.

A massage after a heavy meal is liable to be unpleasant. Therefore, both masseur and patient must see that they come to the massage without a feeling of "heaviness," and their digestive systems busy digesting food. Having said that, they must not come to the treatment hungry and lacking in energy.

The best way is for both of them to eat a light meal about an hour or an hour and a half before the massage.

Before the treatment, the patient must be allowed to lie down for a few minutes to get into the atmosphere, and inhale deep abdominal breaths to relax his body and wind down. During a sexually arousing massage, the partner who is planning the pleasurable experience must see to it that the transition to the intimate stage is smooth and fast, without any need to perform "last-minute preparations" that will suspend the effect of arousal that was achieved during the massage, or cause it to disappear. In an erotic massage, the lighting in the room should be dim, gentle, and pleasant. To this end, a light with a dimmer can be used. Romantic candlelight, or fragrant candles placed at different points around the room, providing sufficient light to see clearly, but still creating an enchanted and romantic atmosphere, is likely to add another dimension of enjoyment to the massage.

Advice for the massage

When we set out to perform a full body massage, we must take into account that this involves a certain amount of physical effort. When the person is not an experienced masseur, he is liable to become tired after twenty minutes or half an hour of massage - and a full body massage (in Shiatsu for Lovers) can take over an hour. For this reason, it is important to decide whether to perform a full body massage, or a partial body massage, which focuses specifically on the sexually arousing points.

Of course, it is important to remember, during an erotic massage, that we can't just go straight to the "strategic areas," because this will not produce a whole lot of pleasure. An erotic massage also has to encompass all the body's surfaces, but, having said that, less time need be devoted to certain parts, so as to avoid fatigue.

In order not to tire out our hands, or to place cold or non-energetic hands on the patient's body, there are a few warm-up movements that we should do before starting the massage: rubbing our hands together vigorously, massaging our fingers with the pad of our thumb by running it along the surface of the hand from top to bottom, and repeating the action with the other hand. Afterward, we should swing our arms, which are hanging loosely at our sides, until they feel warmer, more flexible, and full of energy.

A massage for sexual arousal, combined with Shiatsu pressures

As an example, we present a full body massage that utilizes most of the massage techniques that were mentioned above, while combining massage with pressure on the essential points. In this massage, the couple chose to use a blend of sexually arousing aromatic oils, as well as adding these oils to their bath-water.

Before the massage, Michelle and Dan relaxed in a bath containing stimulating essential oils. They added two drops of jasmine oil, three drops of patchouli, and four drops of ylang ylang to the warm water. After a twenty-minute bath, they dried themselves off, and Michelle lay down on the bed in order to enjoy a slow and pleasurable massage.

Dan began by warming his hands and fingers. A few minutes later, when he felt that his hands were warm and flexible, he smeared a mixture of essential oils (the same ones they had used in the bath) and vegetable oil onto his hands. He placed his hands on Michelle's shoulders; she was lying calm and relaxed on her back on the bed, and Dan covered her whole body with a towel so as to keep her warm, and began to massage her face.

Facial massage is relaxing and calming, and helps the person get into the right frame of mind for an erotic massage. First, Dan placed his hands on either side of Michelle's head. His palms were on her cheeks, and his thumbs were pressing very gently on her forehead. His hands remained in that position for a few moments. Then he began to massage her forehead using long movements. When he reached the pressure point between her eyebrows - a point that greatly relieves pressure and tension, and promotes relaxation and calmness - he placed his finger on the point, applied pressure steadily for about ten seconds, and then gradually and slowly released the pressure, without detaching his finger from the point. He repeated the action three times. He continued massaging Michelle's face gently, while focusing on the pressure point at the top of the bridge of her nose. He applied gradual pressure to this soothing point three times, keeping his finger on the point for about seven seconds, and, without detaching his finger from the point, gradually releasing the pressure. Pressure on this point is excellent at the beginning stages of an erotic massage, because it is very soothing, and helps the person relax and wind down for the rest of the massage.

After applying pressure to this point, Dan continued with the gentle facial massage. He focused on Michelle's lips, drawing his finger over her lips and sketching little circles on their soft surface. Then he concentrated on the pressure point located in the indentation between her upper lip and her nose. This point is also very good at the beginning stages of an erotic massage, since it is very effective in helping the person release tension and pressure, cast off daily worries, and achieve a state of serenity and relaxation. The person can then concentrate fully on the sexual pleasure afforded by the massage. In this way, the point helps intensify the pleasure of the massage and enables the person to concentrate on the sexual enjoyment caused by the erotic massage. Dan applied gentle and gradual pressure on the point, releasing it gradually, without detaching his finger from the point, and repeated the action three times.

After this, he continued the gentle facial massage, combined with stroking, gradually making his way to Michelle's ears. He applied gentle pressure with the pads of his forefingers to the surface below the ear, on the lobe, using touching and pressing movements. He also stroked her lobe, which is very sensitive to caresses, kisses, and oral contact, because of the numerous nerve endings in it. Gentle and pleasant contact with the ear can be very sexually arousing for this reason. Afterward, Dan drew his finger over Michelle's lips. First he sketched light circles with his finger over the upper lip, and then over the lower lip.

Then Dan stood behind Michelle, and gently grasped her nape. He gently pulled his hands one at a time, sliding them upward along her nape, and in a steady movement along the rear surface of her head. He repeated the relaxing movement three times, and the third time, he pulled the roots of her hair lightly, gently separating the strands between his fingers.

Dan progressed to Michelle's shoulders. Still standing behind Michelle, Dan placed his hands on her shoulders, and performed movements of pushing forward, allowing her shoulders to feel the contact with his entire palm. The next step was to perform circular movements on her shoulders by grasping one shoulder in both hands, and turning it three times in a clockwise direction; this was repeated with the other shoulder. After turning her shoulders around a bit, Dan gradually began to knead her arms with steady but gentle movements, and in relaxing pulling movements, until he reached her right hand.

There he concentrated on another important pressure point, which is located on the gap between the thumb and the forefinger, slightly in the direction of the root of the hand, at a distance of a finger-width below the first joint of the forefinger, on the outer part of the hand. Dan applied pressure to the point using the "pinching" technique, placing his forefinger and middle finger on the pad of his thumb, and pressing with his thumb. He pressed on the point three times without detaching his thumb from the point, and then did the same on Michelle's left hand. After repeating the pressure on her left hand, Dan went up her arm using kneading movements, and massaged her shoulders a bit again.

Afterward, he began to slide his fingers, slowly and gently, in the direction of Michelle's chest, sliding his hand along the middle line of her chest. While applying medium pressure, he slid his hands right down her chest and abdomen, until the pubic line. Then he placed both hands on the outer sides of the ribs, and slowly lifted his hands in a circular movement onto the chest itself, while sketching a circular route along the different parts of the chest, from the perimeter of the chest up to the nipples. He performed these movements several times, and then cupped his hands over her chest, placing them in a circular movement on her chest, kneading it and pressing it gently. This is an extremely pleasurable movement, which, besides arousing sexually, is effective in pre-menstrual women who suffer from congestion in the breasts, as it greatly relieves the congestion and discomfort in the breasts.

When he had finished massaging the chest, Dan set about treating Michelle's arms. He performed kneading and massaging movements on her arms, from the upper region to the palm and the fingers, gently pulling the fingers and releasing them. He gently performed the effleurage movements on the chest and abdominal regions, and then performed gentle circular movements on the abdominal region.

While massaging the central abdominal region, Dan focused on the "Pass Organ" pressure point that is located below the navel. This point is generally used for improving sexual functioning and increasing general vigor; during and after the massage, it increases sexual arousal. Dan applied gentle, steady, gradually increasing pressure to it, using his forefinger reinforced by his middle finger, so as to increase the pressure. He kept his finger on the point for about seven seconds, gradually released it without detaching his finger from the point, and repeated the procedure twice more.

After applying pressure to this point, he descended, sliding his hands in gentle circular movements over Michelle's belly to the abdominal slope, and performed gentle tapping movements with his fingers - more fluttering than actually tapping. When he reached the region of the pubic bone, at the bottom of the abdomen, Dan concentrated on the "Crooked Bone" pressure point, which is located at a distance of two finger-widths above the pubic bone. Besides improving and increasing sexual vigor, this point arouses the person almost immediately after being pressed. Dan pressed on the point gently, using his forefinger, gradually increasing the pressure, and keeping his finger on the point for about seven seconds. Then he gradually released the pressure and repeated the action twice more. (Michelle, who was lying relaxed on the bed, took deep, slow breaths. It was obvious from her breathing that Dan had reached the more erogenous areas of her body.) He then descended to the "Middle Extreme" pressure point, the most arousing point during massage and foreplay. He applied gentle, gradual pressure to the point, using the pad of his thumb, until he felt a kind of resistance to his thumb, and at that point he kept his thumb on the point for about ten seconds. Gradually he released the pressure, until his thumb rose to the slightly springy surface of the abdomen. Without detaching his thumb from the point, he repeated the procedure twice more.

At this point, Dan asked Michelle to turn over onto her stomach. Again he smeared oil over his hands, and began to perform warming, circular effleurage movements all over her back, emphasizing her shoulders at the end of the circular, inclusive movement. Afterward, he performed a few kneading movements, using his palm and his fingers, grasping a bit of flesh in his hand. He did this softly, on Michelle's back and shoulders. A few minutes later, he began to perform squeezing movements (petrissage), gently grasping the skin between his thumb and the other fingers, and rolling it up and down, the length of Michelle's back. After spending about twenty minutes treating her back, releasing tension and pain, with Michelle meanwhile enjoying her relaxed and calm state, Dan began to apply pressure to the numerous essential points on her back.

He applied pressure to her lower back region with all his fingers, so as to stimulate simultaneously as many points as possible. He applied stronger pressure to this region than he had to the points in the facial and abdominal regions, paying attention to Michelle's reactions, and ensuring that she could feel the steady pressure, but still find it pleasant. He focused on the regions on each side of the spinal column, while moving his hands from the region that is located a bit below the waist until the crease of her buttocks.

When he had finished applying pressure to these areas, Dan began to knead Michelle's buttocks with strong pressure that released all the tight areas. Afterward, he performed shaking movements that were so releasing that Michelle burst into peels of laughter. The shaking movements of the buttocks greatly relax the muscles and also release mental pressure at the same time. Then Dan spread a bit more oil on his hands, and massaged Michelle's buttocks with circular movements. Very slowly, he moved down to her thighs.

He massaged this region with kneading movements. He grasped her thigh in both hands, with his thumbs on the outer part of her thigh, and descended the length of her thigh using his fingers. Using this form of massage, which encompasses the whole thigh, Dan slowly went down to Michelle's calves. In the thigh region, Dan felt a great deal of tension, most likely stemming from the fact that Michelle spent many hours on her feet at work. Since he did not want to attack the stiff area too aggressively, he performed several circular movements to soften the area, and then began to knead the posterior part of her calf gently, gradually increasing the strength of the pressure.

Then he performed squeezing movements on her calf, grasping it on both sides with his hands, his thumbs pressing on the inner side of her calf, and his palms supporting the vertical squeezing movement by being placed on the outer part of her calf. Dan focused on the pressure point at the base of her calf, at its lowest part, on the inner part of her leg. He applied pressure to the point using the "pinching" technique, keeping his thumb on the point for about seven seconds, and gradually releasing the pressure without detaching his finger from the point. He repeated the procedure three times, and then went on to Michelle's other calf. This point increases sexual vigor and helps the person experience more powerful sensations during sexual activity.

From this point, it was easy to continue to the point on the sole of Michelle's foot, located between the two pads on the sole, slightly in the direction of her big toe. Dan applied increasingly strong pressure to the point - without causing pain, however; he kept his finger on the point for about seven seconds, and gradually released the pressure, without detaching it from the point. He repeated the procedure three times, and then did the same on the other foot.

Using soft, circular movements, Dan went up Michelle's thighs once more, with the aim of reaching the pressure point that is located on the outer side of the thigh. He applied pressure to the point with his hand placed open on the lower part of her buttocks, and his thumb applying gradual pressure to the point. He kept his thumb there for about seven seconds, and then gradually released the pressure, without detaching his thumb from the point. He repeated the procedure three times, and then did the same on her other thigh.

At this point, Dan asked Michelle to lie on her back again. He began to press on her essential points located on the front part of her calves and thighs, starting at the soles of her feet. While he massaged the soles of Michelle's feet, he kneaded them and performed light, circular, relaxing movements. He began to apply pressure to one of the points of the spleen meridian, located above her ankle. This is a very sexually stimulating and invigorating point. Dan used the "pinching" technique to press it, keeping his fingers on the point for about seven seconds, and gradually releasing the pressure. He repeated the procedure three times on each ankle. Then, kneading Michelle's calves, which were more relaxed now after his previous massage, and could tolerate stronger pressure being applied to them, he went up and reached the first essential point located below the knee. This point is very valuable from the point of view of increasing sexual arousal. Dan applied pressure to the point with his forefinger, placing his middle finger on his forefinger to increase the pressure. He applied gradually increasing pressure to the point, kept his finger on the point for a few seconds, and gradually released the pressure. He repeated the procedure twice more. Then he did the same on Michelle's other calf, using kneading movements until he reached the pressure point below her other knee. He repeated the procedure.

While his hands were still grasping Michelle's left leg, he started applying pressure to the point that is used for increasing sexual arousal, located on the inner part of the leg, next to the knee. Dan used the same technique to apply pressure to it for a few seconds, and repeated the procedure twice more. Then he returned to her right leg to apply pressure to the same point there.

Afterward, he began applying the kneading technique to her knee, placing both hands around the outer area of her kneecap, and stimulating the area by means of a series of gentle pressures. After performing this procedure on her left leg, he applied pressure to the point on the outer side of her calf. In order to apply pressure to the point, Dan enclosed Michelle's kneecap in his hand, and used his thumb to apply the pressure. He did this several times, applying gradual pressure to the point, keeping his thumb on the point for about ten seconds, releasing the pressure gradually, and repeating the procedure. Applying pressure to this point is wonderful for improving all aspects of sexual functioning, increasing sexual vigor, and intensifying the sexual experience. Moreover, it is also very soothing, and helps the person feel more open and more prepared mentally and physically for intercourse.

After Dan applied pressure to the same point on the other leg, he went up to the thigh, using pleasant and gentle kneading and pressing movements, until he reached the point next to the thigh. This point is also very effective for increasing sexual arousal and desire. Dan applied gradual pressure, and then released the pressure gradually, repeating the procedure three times on each leg, and moved on to the points on Michelle's upper thigh. In this area, there are numerous points of arousal, and in order to stimulate many of them simultaneously, Dan applied gentle pressure to the inner, front area of her thighs. He stimulated the points, which cause sexual arousal and an increase in sexual desire almost instantaneously, in a variety of ways. First, he caressed the region, then he continued applying steady pressure, and then he massaged the region on each thigh with both hands.

By now, Michelle was feeling extremely aroused sexually, but Dan wouldn't stop. He knew that in order to intensify the experience, he should not stop the treatment at this point. He reached the point located on the pubic bone. After applying pressure to the point several times, still gently stroking the lower part of Michelle's body, he began to focus on the "Conception Vessel" meridian. Applying pressure to these points can constitute a marvelous conclusion to an erotic massage, since, after pressing them, it is possible to begin intercourse, as the degree of arousal is extremely high.

The points of the "Conception Vessel" meridian are the most important in erotic stimulation, so pressure should be applied to them toward the end of the massage. The points are located along the middle line of the lower abdomen. Dan began to apply pressure to the points from the region of the pubic bone, along the middle line, several times to each point, his fingers ascending up to a distance of two finger-widths above the navel. Dan waited to apply pressure to the most important point for sexual stimulation - "The Meeting Point of Feminine Power," which is located between the anus and the genitals, the most powerful point in the degree of stimulation it provides - until the act of intercourse itself.

Now, to conclude the massage, Dan took a long, soft ostrich feather, and began to move it over Michelle's body, focusing on her intimate parts. Michelle, who could not tolerate the slightly ticklish stimulation of the feather, and felt completely aroused and energized, sat up and pulled Dan down to her.

Now they both moved on to the second stage of the erotic massage, in which the massage was just a marginal detail ...

2

Shiatsu for Lovers

Up to this point, you have become familiar with the fundamentals of Shiatsu, the meridians, and the pressure points, and you have learned a great deal about massage (including massage with oils) and pressures. You are now no doubt conversant with the massage and pressure techniques, as well as with the location of the 24 most important "sexual" points in Shiatsu for Lovers.

Although we have presented the subject in general, there is a certain degree of repetition of what has already been written (mainly in the elaboration on the points and the explanation of the erotic massage) in the descriptions of Shiatsu for Lovers.

Now we will move on to the second part of the book, in which we will focus on Shiatsu for Lovers. In this part, we will present the preferred pressures for Shiatsu for Lovers, we will examine several problems and conditions that require special treatment, and we will prepare ourselves for the *pièce de résistance* in the third part, which includes true stories about the wonders of Shiatsu for Lovers.

I will take it for granted that you are familiar with what appeared in the first part of the book, and so from now on I will use mainly the names of the pressures, without going into detail about what has already been described. Every term that appears from here on is explained in the first part of the book.

Unique pressure techniques in Shiatsu for Lovers

In Shiatsu for Lovers, there are two groups of pressure techniques. The first is used during sexual intercourse, and constitutes part of the foreplay and the love-making itself. The second is used to stimulate and accumulate sexual vigor.

In the second technique, the effect is cumulative, as the technique is applied on a daily basis, or several times a week, in order to arouse, balance, and stimulate sexual vitality and vigor, and to solve various sexual problems. This technique is not directly connected to love-making, and can be self-applied, even though it is always preferable for the other member of the couple to apply the pressures.

The Shiatsu pressure techniques from the first group are applied during foreplay, during the sexual act, and after it, and their aim is to be part of the actual love-making. The pressure techniques increase and intensify pleasure during foreplay, and prepare the body for orgasmic release, as well as increase and intensify the orgasm itself.

They are extremely important when the couple's sex life tends to be boring, routine, or unsatisfying, or when there are specific problems in sexual functioning. Later on, we will focus on these points. Remember that there are points whose purpose is to strengthen and arouse sluggish libido, and, conversely, there are points that help to tone down excessive libido.

The advantage of Shiatsu for Lovers is that it does not require physical strength, and every normal person can apply the pressures very easily. In addition to the physical aspect of the pressure points, they contribute to the closeness and psychological awakening of the couple. It is recommended that even if only one member of the couple suffers from any kind of sexual problem, both members pleasure each other with Shiatsu pressures. The effect of mutually applied pressures, whether during intercourse or separately from it, is powerful, extending beyond the actual stimulation of the points. The pressures teach people how to touch each other and discover what kind of touch the other person enjoys and finds pleasurable; it helps people know and accept their own body and that of their partner, and helps eliminate the barriers, inhibitions, and psychological fears that people have concerning sexual relations.

Practicing applying the pressures is very simple, and everyone can do it, alone or in couples. The location of the pressure points is identical in men and in women, but varies relative to the physical build of each individual, depending on size and height.

Locating the points is very easy, but remember that locations such as "four finger-widths" or "a palm's length" refer to the *patient's* body - that is, the person who is receiving the Shiatsu. Therefore, when you set out to apply pressures to your partner, you must measure the points *according to the width or length of his/her fingers.*

The strength of the pressure to be applied is medium - neither too strong nor too weak - and you should press until just before it hurts; however, you must not reach the point of pain. In the case of a person who is overweight, the pressure should be slightly greater, in order to reach the points. In the case of an especially thin person, the pressure should be lighter and more superficial. As a person gets older, the sensitivity of his nerves in certain places diminishes, which means that these points need greater stimulation. You should not press too hard, but you should press for *a longer time* in order to ensure the correct and optimal stimulation of the point.

The pressures

In Shiatsu for Lovers, we mainly use the four pressures that are detailed here, as well as a small or large variety of massage techniques that precede or combine with the pressures.

It is a good idea to practice these pressures - especially on oneself, in order to feel the sensation and learn the degree of strength necessary for each pressure.

Thumb pressure: The most convenient and effective form of pressure is that applied with the thumb. By means of this pressure, it is possible to use a great deal of strength, and to press deeply into the flesh.

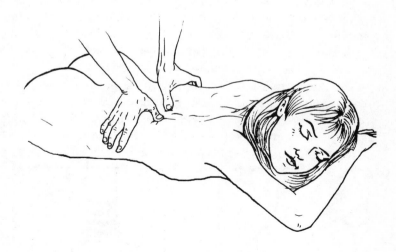

It is important to ensure that your fingernails are short before applying the pressure, since, during a vertical thumb pressure, which is the most effective, long fingernails are liable to hurt your partner.

Finger pressure: Another form of pressure is that applied with the forefinger or middle finger. Since the pressure applied by these fingers is not great, you can press with your forefinger while reinforcing it with your middle finger, which is pressing on the top joint of the forefinger.

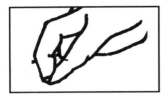 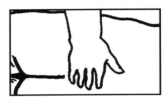

"Pinching" pressure: In certain regions of the body, it is easier to apply pinching pressure. This does not mean actual pinching with the fingers, but rather a "pinch" with the whole palm, or with some of the fingers, in order to grasp the place where the point is located.

This technique can be applied to a particular point in order to increase the thumb pressure, or to press more steadily with the thumb. In such a case, most of the strength of the pressure must be transferred to the thumb.

It is preferable to use this technique only in cases where it

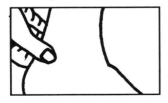 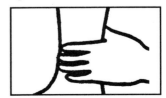

is not possible to use only the thumb - for instance, when pressing the sides of the ankle, or certain points on the palm. In any case, the pressure is applied by the thumb, which is the main "presser" in this technique, while the fingers serve as counter-supports.

Applying pressure using the pads of the palms: This pressure is used when you need to press on a larger area, on two or more points simultaneously, or on an area that contains a large number of points very close to one another.

In this technique, your palms are placed parallel to each other on the center of the area, and the pressure of your body is channeled into the pads of the palms. This form of pressure creates a strong, steady pressure on the points.

The pressures must be applied gradually, up to just *before* the point where the person begins to feel a little pain. This is

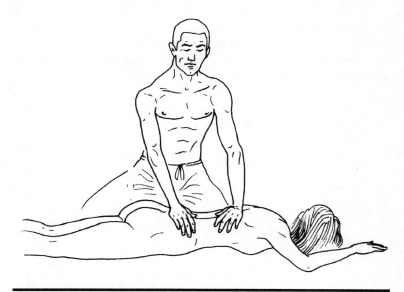

when the pressure should cease, and the finger should be held on the point for between five and ten seconds.

After this, the pressure exerted by the finger should be gradually reduced, until the finger is touching the point without any pressure.

Remember that you must not jab the point suddenly and quickly, or release the finger abruptly. Everything should be done slowly and gradually. When your finger is touching the point without pressure, you must wait about five seconds, and then, without detaching it from the point, gradually begin to apply pressure again. This procedure should generally be repeated three times before moving on to the next point.

During the pressure, do not rotate your finger or thumb, or "dig" with them, or perform massaging movements. The pressure must be direct and steady.

We will now go on to a survey of the problems and conditions in which Shiatsu for Lovers - applying pressure to certain points - helps provide relief, healing, and solutions to problems in the sexual realm that are widespread among men and women.

Problems, diseases, and treatment situations

Relieving menstrual cramps and pains

The cramps and other pains and symptoms that accompany the monthly period can be very effectively relieved by applying Shiatsu pressures. Because of their importance, we will elaborate on all eight central points for this situation.

**Please note that from here on,
the numbers in square brackets relate to the list of points
in the first part of the book.**

The pressure point below the knee, slightly toward the inner side of the leg [9]: Apply pressure gradually with your thumb, keep it on the point for between five and ten seconds, then gradually release the pressure. Repeat this procedure at least three times.

The pressure point at the base of the calf, on the inner part of the leg [11]: It is easier to press this point using "pinching" pressure, but you can also press it with your forefinger reinforced by your middle finger on its upper joint. Apply the pressure gradually, keep your finger on the point for about seven seconds, and then release the pressure gradually. Without detaching your finger from the point, repeat this procedure at least three times.

The pressure point above the knee, toward the inner side of the leg [12]: This pressure is easy to apply if you enclose your partner's knee in your palm and apply gradual pressure with your thumb, keep it on the point for seven to ten seconds, then gradually releasing the pressure. Without detaching your thumb from the point, repeat the procedure three to five times.

The pressure point on the outer part of the thigh [13]: Pressure should be applied to this point by someone else, while the woman who is receiving the treatment is standing. Gradual pressure is applied to the point with the thumb, keeping it there for about seven seconds, and gradually releasing the pressure. Without detaching the thumb from the point, this procedure is repeated at least three times.

The "Intersection of the Three Yins" point [1]: You should use the "pinching" technique, with your thumb placed on the point, and your fingers serving as supports. Apply pressure gradually, from light to medium, and keep your thumb on the point for about seven seconds. Release the pressure gradually, and, without detaching your thumb from the point, repeat the procedure at least three times.

The "Sea of Blood" point [2]: Pressure on this point is applied when the woman is seated on a chair, and her partner covers her kneecap with his hand. The point is located under his thumb, when he is seated in the floor (or on a cushion) in front of her. Pressure should be applied gradually to the point, the thumb should be kept on the point for about ten seconds, and then the pressure should be released gradually. Without detaching the thumb from the point, this procedure should be repeated at least three times.

The "Original Chi" point [3]: This point is located in the middle of the abdomen. Using the thumb or forefinger, apply pressure gradually but gently, and keep your finger on the point for five to ten seconds. Gradually release the pressure, and, without detaching your finger from the point, repeat the procedure about three times.

The "Walking Three Miles" point [4]: This point is

located at a distance of four finger-widths below the kneecap. With your fingers enveloping the kneecap, apply gradual pressure with your thumb, and gradually release. Repeat the procedure at least three times. This point is the most important one, and is also used for general strengthening.

In order to obtain the optimal results in relieving menstrual pains and cramps as well as emotional imbalance, and so on, these pressures should be applied on a daily basis (during the period), at least three times on each point. It is best to apply pressure to all the points, but you can make do with some of them only.

Points for relieving menopausal symptoms

Shiatsu pressure has been shown to be extremely effective in relieving menopausal symptoms such as hot and cold flashes, backaches, tremors, sudden feelings of exhaustion, and so on. In addition, these pressures relieve the emotional aspects of menopause to a great extent.

The points that are used for relieving menopausal symptoms are:

The point on the bridge of the nose, between the eyebrows [14] (only one in the body).

The point on the sole of the foot, between the two balls of the foot, slightly toward the big toe [15]. Pressure should be applied to both feet.

Points for relieving the symptoms of mid-life crisis in men

The mid-life crisis in men may manifest itself in mental and emotional symptoms, rather than physical ones. In general, this period occurs in men between the ages of 45 and 55. The condition may be expressed in a feeling of general disappointment in the man's status in life (a feeling of unfulfilled potential from the business, intellectual or economic point of view, a feeling of having wasted his life on the wrong career, a lack of interest in or boredom with life, dissatisfaction with his social circle, a feeling of loneliness, and so on).

This is liable to create a situation in which the importance of the man's sex life deteriorates as a result of a loss of interest; this affects sexual intercourse itself, and leads to a destructive vicious circle. Sometimes this situation leads to a quest for new extramarital sexual excitement, which causes guilt feelings.

It is possible to alleviate this mental and psychological condition by applying Shiatsu for Lovers. If the man's partner (wife) is the one who is applying the pressure, an additional advantage is gained - that of bringing the couple closer together. The man is given a good and encouraging feeling of caring, touch and softness - things for which he may not know how to express his need. Besides the actual Shiatsu pressures, these things also help him to overcome the mid-life crisis.

Pressure is applied mainly to the general strengthening points, such as the "Original Chi" point [3], which is located in the center of the abdomen. This point should be pressed with the thumb, or with the forefinger reinforced by the middle finger to increase pressure. The pressure is applied gradually, and the finger is kept on the point for about ten seconds, while the man takes deep breaths that fill the hollow of his stomach. The pressure is then gradually released. It is very important not to detach the finger from the point abruptly, but rather to release the pressure slowly and gradually. This procedure should be repeated at least three times, without detaching the finger from the point.

The second point is the "Walking Three Miles" point [4], which is located at a distance of four finger-widths below the kneecap. The point should be pressed in the same way as the "Original Chi" point. The procedure should be repeated at least three times.

In addition to these points, the rest of the points that are pressed during love play are also likely to relieve symptoms of the mid-life crisis.

Frigidity

This difficult problem, which characterizes many women, tends to be divided into two main types when diagnosed: First, when the woman does not feel any sexual arousal at all during sexual intercourse; and second, when there is sexual arousal, but it fades at a certain point, and she does not reach orgasm.

The first thing that the woman must do is determine for herself whether she really is frigid. If she feels pleasure during sexual intercourse, feels satisfied and reaches orgasm, regardless of its intensity, she is not frigid. She has to decide for herself to be aware of her sensations during intercourse. No matter how understanding and aware her partner is, he cannot determine this.

All the sexual arousal points that are used in Shiatsu for

Lovers are known to have a significant effect on this problem, and by persistent application of pressure to these points, good results can be achieved.

Out of points **5, 6, 7, 8, 10, 11, 16, 17, 18, 19, 20, 21, 22,** and **23,** five to eight should be chosen, and pressure applied to them twice a day for a few weeks.

Besides the sexual arousal points, there are specific meridians that can also lead to good results when pressure is applied to them: The stomach meridian, next to the pubic bone, and below the knee; the liver meridian, next to the thigh; the spleen meridian, on the inner side of the leg next to the knee; and a point on the meridian above the ankle. (The latter treatment belongs to Shiatsu, Zen Shiatsu, and meridian exercises, and are not described in this book.)

Preferred sexual arousal points

In Shiatsu for Lovers, there are four main arousal zones: the back, the lower abdomen and the perineum, the upper thigh, and the ear.

The back

Around the sacrum - the big bone at the base of the spinal column - there are a number of nerves that supply energy to the reproductive organs. Those nerves, together with the nerves in the region of the lower back, control almost all the vital functions of the lower part of the body, such as erection, sexual intercourse, and so on. It is possible to stimulate 12 to 15 nerves simultaneously with each application of pressure. The pressure can be applied with all the fingers simultaneously or with the whole hand.

Pressure is applied gradually, from light to medium, in the areas described in point number **19**.

The "Conception Vessel One" point or perineum
The perineum is the gap between the genitals and the anus in both sexes. The perineal point is located on the "Conception Vessel" meridian **[8]**, and is in fact the first point on the meridian.

The perineal point is one of the most important points for erotic stimulation and for treating various kinds of sexual problems.

The meridian continues along the center line of the lower abdomen. All five points of this meridian are extremely important for sexual arousal, and they can be stimulated during foreplay, or for strengthening and balancing the sexual system on a daily basis. The points start at the groin bone, continue up along the center line, and get to about two finger-widths above the navel. These points are close together and are even on top of other points that are used in Shiatsu for Lovers (see comment on page 62).

Points on the upper thigh
The points on the thighs - mainly in the front part - are very numerous, and are spread over a broad surface, and it is difficult to miss them when gentle pressure is applied to the inner and frontal region of the thighs. They can be stimulated in any way: by constant pressure, by stroking, and by massage. The main point is number **20**, but **13** and **17** also play a role.

Points on the ear

There are numerous nerves on the ear [21]. One of them is the vagus, which runs from the base of the brain along the entire length of the body, sending signals to many other nerves, and playing a role in the operation of the autonomic nervous system. The autonomic nervous system, which oversees many involuntary actions in the body, also plays a part in various actions of the sexual and reproductive systems. This means that various ways of touching the ear, such as nibbling, kissing, sucking, or touching, cause sexual arousal, and are effective during love play.

Pressure on the part of the lobe that is parallel to the temple is likely to be effective in many situations of sexual dysfunction, and in a variety of sexual disorders. Applied on a daily basis, it will also increase the libido generally.

"Distant" points for treating sexual problems

Pressure is applied to these points on a daily basis in order to improve all aspects of sexual function, and to increase potency. During intercourse, they also serve to intensify the sexual experience. These points strengthen the entire body.

The points are called "distant" because they are located far from the genitals. They can be used in daily practice in situations in which it is impossible to apply pressure to the more "intimate" points - for example, while riding on the bus - or when the person is reluctant to indulge in too close a relationship. Of course, it is possible to include pressure on these points in every stage of Shiatsu for Lovers.

The pressure point on the hand [22]: It is easy to apply "pinching" pressure to this point by placing the forefinger on the pad of the thumb, and pressing the point with the thumb. The point is located parallel to the bone, not on it.

Many people feel pain in this point, indicating a certain general lack of balance in the body, so gentle pressure should be applied at first. Applying pressure on a daily basis will gradually cause the pain to decrease, while generally strengthening and balancing the body. This point should be pressed at least three times on both hands. Pressure is applied gradually for five to ten seconds, and then gradually released, without detaching the thumb from the point; then pressure is applied gradually again.

The pressure point on the outer side of the calf [11]: This region is also likely to hurt a bit, so gentle pressure should be applied at first.

The pressure point at the bottom of the calf [12], on the inner side of the leg: Pressure can be applied to the point using the thumb, or by "pinching," placing the thumb on the point and using it to apply most of the pressure.

The Love Points - points that are "close"

Applying pressure to these points is actually meant for anyone who is not fully aroused by foreplay - poor erection, vaginal dryness, and so on. The points are called "close" both because they are located close to the genitals, and because pressure should be applied to them just before intercourse.

As we mentioned, besides being used on a daily basis for increasing sexual potency and improving sexual function, these points are considered the most arousing during foreplay.

The "Pass Organ" point [15]: Pressure can be applied to it with the thumb, the forefinger, or the forefinger reinforced by the middle finger in order to increase the pressure. Pressure should be applied gently and gradually, keeping the finger on the point for five to ten seconds. The finger is then released gradually, but not detached from the point, and then the pressure is applied again. This procedure should be repeated three to five times.

The "Middle Extreme" point [6]: This point should also be pressed gently, using the same techniques as for the "Pass Organ" point above, keeping the finger on the point for about seven seconds. The finger is then released gradually, but not detached from the point, and the pressure is applied again. This procedure should be repeated at least three times.

The "Crooked Bone" point [7]: This point is located at a distance of two finger-widths above the "Middle Extreme" point. This point should be pressed using the same techniques as for the "Pass Organ" and "Middle Extreme" points above, keeping the finger on the point for five to ten seconds. This procedure should be repeated at least three times.

Points for relieving extreme tension (that spoils sexual intercourse)

In order to derive pleasure from sexual activity and enjoyment from sexual intercourse, both partners must be relaxed, calm, and focused on the lovemaking and intercourse. The numerous incidences of extreme tension in everyday life constitute a significant and widespread factor in the many problems that arise during sex.

Many cases of secondary impotence (that is, impotence that has no medical or physiological origin), frigidity (that does not derive from medical or physiological causes), premature ejaculation, non-ejaculation or delayed ejaculation, pains during intercourse because of a psychological lack of preparedness for the act, agitation during intercourse, delayed orgasm, and many other problems that come to the fore in the sex lives of both men and women alike, are caused or exacerbated by anxieties, agitation, and tension during foreplay and intercourse.

The contribution of Shiatsu for Lovers to the alleviation of tension and agitation is extremely significant, and, as a result, its contribution to relieving and even solving many problems connected to the sexual act is appreciable.

Pressure should be applied to these points in any situation in which the person feels that he is becoming agitated, tense or anxious.

These situations can range from driving (pressure should be applied to the points before getting into the car in the morning, and not while driving, of course - but you can apply pressure to them while stuck in traffic jams or at traffic lights - it's even advisable to do so!), to an exam context, a stressful meeting, public speaking, and so on. Of course, pressure should be applied before intercourse in order to promote calmness and relaxation, and feel as detached as possible from everyday hassles and difficulties; in order to achieve greater and more significant satisfaction and pleasure, and to function in the optimal way before, during, and after intercourse.

The points that are presented below even help in lowering high blood pressure, and in this way alleviate problems in sexual function (especially in men) that stem from hypertension. The points are:

The point on the outer side of the calf [11]: Remember that pressure on this area is liable to hurt a bit, mainly in cases of imbalance and extreme, ongoing agitation, so that gentle pressure should be applied at first. After applying pressure for some time, and balance has gradually been restored and tension released, there will be less pain during the application of pressure, and then greater pressure can be applied to the point. This pressure should be applied while the person is seated, with the "presser's" palm enveloping the person's knee, and the thumb applying pressure to the point. The procedure should be repeated at least three times, applying gradual pressure, keeping the finger on the point for five to ten seconds, and releasing the pressure gradually.

The pressure point between the eyebrows [23]: Pressure can be applied to this point with the thumb, but it is easier to apply pressure with the forefinger or middle finger. There is no need to use a lot of strength while pressing, as there isn't a large mass of tissue to penetrate. Pressure can be applied with the forefinger reinforced by the middle finger in order to increase the pressure. Gradual pressure is applied, keeping your finger on the point for about seven seconds, and then gradually releasing the pressure, without detaching your finger from the point. The procedure is repeated at least three times. This is a superb point for dispelling tension, agitation, and pressure, and is also effective in cases of headaches.

The pressure point between the upper lip and the nose [24]: Gentle pressure should be applied to it gradually, never strong pressure (that is, you should never reach a situation in which pressure is applied to the front teeth that lie below this point). This procedure of gradual pressure and gradual release should be repeated at least three times without detaching the finger from the point. The person should take deep breaths during the pressure. This point, besides its contribution to relaxation and the release of tension, is also known as a point that stimulates facial beauty and the skin.

As you can see, it is amazingly simple to apply pressure to these points. There is no limit to the frequency or to the number of times per day that they can be pressed, and the procedure can be performed in any place and at any time. Despite their simplicity and their convenient location, they are marvelous for dispelling tension. It is a good idea to apply pressure to them when you get up in the morning, and before going to sleep at night. Applying pressure to these points while lying down, feeling comfortable, and taking deep breaths and relaxing the body will enhance sexual vigor and the pleasure during sexual intercourse and the ability to concentrate on sexual enjoyment, as well as increase the body's vitality.

3

Stories of Shiatsu for Lovers

The following examples are taken from patients' files, in which Shiatsu for Lovers was used to solve various sexual problems. The patients (and their partners) learned the massage and pressure methods, as well as the importance of the various pressure points, applied what they had learned, and came back to report. (The numbers in square brackets represent the numbers of the points as they appear in the list in the first part of the book, pages 58-86.)

Pains during penetration

I recall the case of Melanie and Allan, a young couple who consulted with me because of the considerable pain that Melanie experienced during sex - during penetration, to be precise. They arrived together, and displayed equal and honest willingness to deal with the problem. Since they had already undergone several examinations and treatments for their predicament, they had no difficulty describing it to me in minute detail.

Melanie and Allan had been married for three years. From the very first time they had had sex, and then throughout the course of their marriage, Melanie suffered from significant vaginal pains each time Allan tried to penetrate her. Melanie explained that she felt aroused, and was ready for penetration - even desired it - but since it caused her pain every time, she had begun to develop a psychological fear of it, which, of course, intensified the pain.

The situation was extremely frustrating for both of them, and Allan confessed that at a certain point, he felt as if Melanie no longer wanted or desired him. Even though there was no rational basis for this, it was one of the feelings he experienced as a result of their difficulties in having intercourse. This feeling caused his libido to drop, and frequently, even though he desired Melanie, he preferred to abstain in order to avoid getting into the physically and psychologically painful situation of what he interpreted deep down as "rejection." (While he frequently masturbated *alone*, the two of them did not tackle the problem by means of oral sex, mutual masturbation, and so on.)

Melanie told me that Allan had been the first man she had

had sex with, as she came from quite a conservative family. She had met him while she was in high school, and had decided to marry him at the age of 19. She admitted that she had been disappointed in their wedding night. Although Allan had pleasured her and made her feel good, and she loved and desired him with all her heart, the pain that she had experienced during penetration had turned the whole thing into a trauma for her, and she just couldn't understand how, when she so desired Allan, she was unable to enjoy it when he penetrated her. Friends in whom Melanie had confided calmed her down and told her that the pain would soon pass. But it hadn't. On the contrary - it even increased somewhat when she began to experience psychological fear as a result of the unsuccessful attempts at intercourse.

Luckily for them, their conjugal life was filled with love and understanding, and they tried to relate to the problem tolerantly, and put it into the correct perspective. In the beginning, Allan thought that the problem stemmed from insufficient sexual stimulation, so he tried different methods and foreplay techniques to increase stimulation before penetration. While he did in fact get Melanie to reach orgasm without penetration, none of his attempts to solve the problem succeeded.

After about a year, they began to undergo various gynecological examinations and treatments. Melanie underwent numerous exhausting tests to see whether the source of the problem was physiological. Both of their genitals were of average size, so this was not a physiological problem. When it became clear that Melanie wasn't suffering from a physiological problem, nor did she have any psychological problem concerning either her body or sexual intercourse per se, the couple was left with no solution to the problem. They decided to try (sexual) Shiatsu. Perhaps this would help them.

It was recommended that Melanie and Allan try Shiatsu for Lovers in order to help decrease the pain that Melanie experienced during penetration, and ultimately to eliminate it altogether. Melanie was told to focus daily on the points that promote relaxation and reduce tension, preferably with Allan's help and participation. The points were:

The point on the outer side of the calf [11]: At the beginning of the pressure application, the point should be pressed rather gently, and gradually, after the pressure has been applied to the point for a period of time, it can be increased. Melanie could apply the pressure herself, but it was better for Allan to do so. The way to apply pressure is by using the thumb to exert steady and gradual pressure, keeping the thumb on the point for about seven seconds, and releasing the pressure gradually. This procedure was to be repeated at least three times, several times a day. Most importantly, it was to be performed a little while before having sex.

The pressure point between the eyebrows [23]: Melanie was advised to apply pressure to this point several times a day, using her forefinger reinforced by her middle finger. The pressure was to be gentle but steady, and gradual, keeping the finger on the point for about seven seconds, and gradually releasing the pressure without detaching the finger from the point. This procedure was to be repeated at least three times each session.

The pressure point between the upper lip and the nose [24]: Pressure was to be applied gently and gradually, but never too strongly. Melanie was to repeat this procedure at least three times, without detaching her finger from the point.

While pressing, she was to pay attention to her breathing, and take deep, slow, calm breaths.

Before having sex, the couple was advised to take a long, warm, fragrant bath together, in order to relax physically and emotionally. While in the bath, they were to soap each other, and pay attention to each other's body. They should concentrate especially on the perineal point, which is located between the anus and the genitals in both males and females. Before touching this point, they were to focus on the "Conception Vessel" points [8], which are very helpful both in sexual arousal and for strengthening and balancing the sexual system. Pressure was to also be applied gently and gradually to these points during foreplay, keeping the finger on the points for five to ten seconds. These points could be caressed or stimulated - by the tongue, for instance.

After the bath, Melanie and Allan were to dry each other and rub aromatic oil or lavender water all over their bodies and around the genitals, the perineal point, the lower back, and the thighs. Rubbing in the oil or lavender water soothes the body, and, simultaneously - especially when the couple do this to each other - stimulates the senses, causes an increased flow of blood to the sexual regions, arouses the nervous system, and increases the sensitivity of the skin in anticipation of touch.

When both members of the couple were ready, it was time to get into bed. Although the bath, the drying, the pressures and the touching stimulate and arouse desire, true passion must be trapped, and kept on a "back burner," so that it will erupt suddenly. As anticipation intensifies passion, it would promote Melanie's physical and psychological readiness for penetration.

Because of the fears she had been nursing for such a long

time, she had to be completely relaxed, and totally focused on enjoyment. She had to remember that she was the one who had to tell Allan when she was ready for penetration, while Allan had to be patient. They were to caress each other with their hands, stimulating and massaging the different parts of their bodies.

There are many points that contribute to the arousal of the sexual stimulus and to the intensification of passion on the earlobes, neck, face, elbows, and knees. Gentle pressure should be applied to these points - not in a technical way, but rather as part of love play.

During this play, Allan was to focus on applying pressure to the region of Melanie's lower back, around the sacral bone (the large bone at the base of the spinal column) [19]. In this region, there are several nerves that provide energy to the reproductive organs, and applying pressure to them was likely to release the tension in the area of Melanie's sexual system, and help to bring release and physical relaxation to those areas, thus facilitating penetration and preventing pain. As Melanie was slender and delicate in build, light to medium pressure was applied to the points on her back with all the fingers. These points were also to be massaged - along with the whole lower back region - using circular, delicate or slightly stronger movements, according to how Melanie felt.

After focusing on the Shiatsu points on the lower back, Allan was to get to the points on the thighs [20], which are located mainly in the front. In this region, there are numerous points, and almost every pressure applied in the inner and front region of the thighs would touch one of Melanie's arousal points. These points can be aroused in any manner - by constant pressure, by caressing, by massaging, or by tongue or mouth contact.

After focusing on these points, Allan gradually had to reach the points located on Melanie's "Conception Vessel" meridian [8], which she knew from the bath. They start at the pubic bone, and go up to above the navel. After applying light pressure to these points and arousing them, he could begin applying pressure to the "love points" - the points that are located close to the genitals (see further on). Besides the inclusion of these points in foreplay in order to stimulate and arouse before intercourse, Melanie was advised to apply pressures to these areas during her daily sessions, in order to strengthen her sexual vitality and improve her sexual functioning.

Allan was to apply the pressure to Melanie, while Melanie did the same for Allan (even if he didn't need it), since applying pressure to one's partner's points, whether during foreplay or in a daily session, strengthens the relationship between the couple and familiarizes them with each other's body, with the kind of touch each one likes, and with his or her arousal points.

There are three of these points, which are located relatively close to the genitals, and for this reason, applying pressure to them serves a dual purpose: arousal of the points by Shiatsu pressure, and sexual stimulation and arousal as a result of the proximity of the genitals. (See comment on page 62.)

The first point to which pressure should be applied is the "Crooked Bone" point [7]. Using the thumb, the forefinger or the middle finger, pressure should be applied to it steadily, but not too heavily. Since Melanie's body was a little fuller in the abdominal region, Allan had to apply the pressure a bit more deeply, by reinforcing the pressure of his forefinger on the point with his middle finger, and pressing slowly but forcefully, applying gradual pressure to the point, and keeping his finger on it for about ten seconds, while Melanie took slow, deep breaths. Then he gradually released the pressure. Pressure could be applied to this point several times, according to how Melanie felt. (Melanie was told to apply pressure herself to this point during her daily sessions, but it was preferable for Allan to do it as well. Allan was also likely to be helped by applying pressure to this point.)

The second point is the "Pass Organ" point [5], which is located in the center of the abdomen. Pressure can be applied to it with the thumb or the forefinger reinforced by the middle finger, in order to increase the pressure. Pressure should be applied gradually to the point at least three times (more frequently during daily sessions), keeping the finger on the point for about seven seconds. The pressure is then gradually released, without detaching the finger from the point. The whole procedure is repeated.

The third point is the "Middle Extreme" point [6], which is located on the slope of the abdomen. Pressure should also be applied to this point on a daily basis, in the same way as the "Pass Organ" point.

It is important to remember that during foreplay, it is neither necessary nor desirable to apply the pressure in a technical, matter-of-fact way, as during daily sessions, but rather to incorporate it into the foreplay, and to precede the application of pressure on the point with caresses and light, pleasant touches. The partners should be physically close to each other, in a reclining or comfortable sitting position, which are some of the pre-coital positions. In this way, treatment of points 8, 7, 5, and 6 can be done consecutively, including massage, pressure, caresses, and so on.

Gradually, when both partners felt more aroused and

excited, the perineal point ("The Point of The Meeting of Feminine Power") [8], which is located between the genitals and the anus, was to be reached. The pressure applied to this point must be gentle but steady, and part of the sex play itself - arousing and stimulating - and Melanie and Allan were to apply this pressure to each other.

Frequently, after touching and caressing this point, and applying pressure to it, both partners feel ready for intercourse. It was important for Melanie to be tuned in to her emotions and physical feelings, and indicate to Allan the correct and appropriate moment for penetration, which was to be performed slowly and gently.

Other positions that could make actual penetration easier for Melanie - in addition to her being calm and aroused by pressures that Allan applied - were lying on her back with a cushion under her buttocks, or her "calling the tune" by straddling Allan (lying on his back), and controlling the penetration according to how she felt.

Other points that the couple were advised to press on a daily basis and incorporate into foreplay, intercourse, and after intercourse, were the "distant" points for improving sexual function, and for increasing sexual vitality.

The first of these points is located on the hand [22]. It is easy to apply "pinching" pressure to this spot. At the beginning of the session, very gentle pressure should be applied, as this point is liable to hurt a bit because of the general state of imbalance in the body. After pressure has been applied to the point for some time, it is possible and desirable to increase it gradually. Each time, the point on *both* hands should be pressed at least three times each. Gradual pressure should be applied, keeping the finger on the point for five to ten seconds, releasing the pressure gradually, and then, without detaching the finger from the point, repeating the procedure by applying gradual pressure.

The second of the distant points is located on the calf [11]. This pressure point tends to be a bit painful when there is a state of imbalance in the body, which means that Allan had to remember to apply gentle pressure to it when he performed Shiatsu for Lovers on Melanie, and gradually, after some time, increase the pressure.

The third point is located at the base of the calf [10]. Pressure was to be applied gradually to the point with the thumb, or by "pinching," applying gradual pressure, keeping the thumb on the point for five to ten seconds, and then gradually releasing the pressure without detaching the thumb from the point. This procedure was to be repeated at least three times each session. However, if this pressure is applied during foreplay, the number of times and the mode of pressing are more flexible, and depend on the couple.

During foreplay and even during intercourse itself, attention should be paid to the ear and the earlobe, as nibbles, kisses, sucking, and even nibbles all intensify sexual arousal and passion during love play. Pressure should be applied to the part of the earlobe that is parallel to the temple, as this point is known for its great effectiveness in various situations of sexual dysfunction and all kinds of sexual problems, and even contributes to the increase of sexual desire in general by means of daily pressing sessions, as well as during love-making in particular.

Melanie and Allan practiced applying these pressures over a period of several months - both in daily sessions (during which Melanie applied them to herself some of the time, and Allan worked with her some of the time), and also in bed, during love-making, foreplay, and intercourse. The first noticeable progress made by Melanie was her gradual release from the tension and fear that accompanied the sexual act and penetration - feelings that she had "nurtured" and magnified as a result of many unpleasant experiences. Melanie discovered that when the barriers of fear were gradually released, the pain diminished, and sexual enjoyment increased appreciably, even though during the first months she still experienced vaginal pain during penetration. This pain gradually diminished, until Melanie reached the point, about six months later, that the occurrence of the pain was extremely rare.

The couple's sexual desire increased enormously, and their sexual relations became more interesting and satisfying. Now, on the rare occasions that Melanie did experience pain, it was mild and totally tolerable, and did not detract from her sexual pleasure. The couple did not stop their daily sessions, so there was every chance that within another few months, the pain that had caused Melanie so much suffering for so long would be a thing of the past.

Impotence, agitation and mid-life crisis

Todd, a 52-year-old managing director of a large diamond company, came to me with his wife, Jodi, for treatment, after suffering from a very disturbing problem for a long time. Todd and Jodi had been married for over 25 years, and had three grown children. For most of their married life, their sexual relations had been enjoyable and satisfying. Three years previously, however, Todd began to suffer from an incomplete erection, a condition which gradually worsened, until he failed to reach an erection altogether - that is, he became impotent. Todd underwent a number of medical examinations, but they revealed that his general health was good, and he was not suffering from any significant physical problem. However, as he explained, the problem - which he perceived as shameful, secret and extremely harmful to his masculinity - had many serious psychological effects. Jodi was suffering from the whole business just as much as Todd was.

At a certain point, after it became clear that he was suffering from a problem with his erection, Todd began to blame Jodi, as a kind of act of denial. He claimed that their sex life had become boring, that she no longer made any effort to stimulate him, and - during one of their rows, which resulted from the state of perpetual frustration that he was in because of his sexual inadequacy - he even threw the bombshell that "he needed new stimulation," and that it was obvious that "she no longer turned him on sexually." After he realized how much anguish these accusations caused Jodi, he admitted that they were not true. Jodi, a mature woman in her late forties, was a shapely and well-groomed woman who had always taken a lot of trouble with her appearance, and was considered very attractive and sexy by one and all. For her part, Jodi tried everything to arouse Todd's desire for her, from sexy lingerie to various sex games and accessories. However, her efforts failed to restore Todd's potency, and only caused him greater frustration. He admitted that he was attracted to Jodi, as he always had been during their marriage, and was dying to have sex with her, but he just couldn't.

Another fear that went hand-in-hand with his problem was that she would finally get sick and tired of him, even though he tried to satisfy her using other methods, and succeeded in doing so. He was afraid that her sexual interest in him would wane.

During the course of a lengthy conversation with Todd and Jodi, I tried to pinpoint the onset of the problem. In an attempt to reconstruct the first instances when he had not succeeded in reaching a full erection, Todd recalled that they had coincided exactly with the time he had run into financial difficulties as a result of a serious crisis in the diamond market. He related that he had made every effort to conceal his financial troubles from his family, and, in fact, Jodi knew nothing about the major crisis Todd was experiencing until long after he had managed to get his business back on an even keel. He added that at the time he was extremely tense and anxious, his blood pressure had risen, he suffered from headaches, and he was incessantly tormented by thoughts of the future of the company and of his family.

It was no wonder he had problems in his sexual performance during intercourse. In order to have enjoyable and satisfying sex, both members of the couple must be calm, relaxed, and totally involved in the love-making. It is not possible to have sex under conditions of stress, anxiety and worry.

The first times Todd failed to reach a full erection became a vicious circle that not only undermined his sexual confidence, but also caused a serious deterioration in his condition - until he was totally impotent (although he could get an erection when he masturbated on his own). His problem of impotence had been compounded by the mid-life crisis he had undergone in a disturbing form. He said that since his eldest son had left home, and his second son had enlisted, he felt less and less "needed" and important at home; occasionally he had the feeling that his only function was to bring in the bacon, nothing more.

Jodi, who was aware of his state of mind and feelings, did everything in her power to express her love for him, but Todd found it difficult to accept her declarations of love because of the feeling of "free fall" that preoccupied him disproportionately. He was filled with anxiety that he would never have an erection again, and admitted that the thought of "doing it with other women" had occurred to him. He had refrained from doing so, however, out of love for Jodi and fidelity to her. His attitude was, "If I can't satisfy my wife fully, and I can't have an erection, what kind of man am I?" His fears of aging only increased his suffering.

A heavy load was removed from Todd's shoulders when he succeeded in identifying and understanding the basic reason for his impotence. He understood that his condition had been exacerbated and aggravated by the anxiety that beset him after his first failures to reach a full erection (because of his worries and tension). Now he began to believe and hope that it was in fact possible to turn the situation around, and that there was a good chance that his sexual performance would return to normal, as it had been in the past.

When treating Todd's secondary impotence problem, a combination of four factors had to be treated together, each of which was significant in Todd's inability to have an erection. These factors were: (i) The symptoms of the mid-life crisis, which Todd was experiencing; (ii) his agitation and anxiety when he wanted to have sex, as a result of his previous failures; (iii) reinforcement and increase of his vitality in general, and his sexual vitality in particular; (iv) increasing his libido, which had decreased in general and during sexual intercourse in particular.

In order to treat this combination of factors, the couple received the following recommendations for treatment:

First of all, Todd was to perform the following daily practice on Shiatsu points in order to relieve the symptoms of the mid-life crisis. These points would relieve both the physical symptoms and the emotional aspects of the mid-life crisis that Todd was going through rather badly. Every day for at least two months (and after that once every two or three days), Todd was to apply pressure to the following points:

The pressure point located just above the bridge of the nose [14]: Todd was to apply pressure to this point using his forefinger. The pressure should not be too strong. He was to keep his finger on the point for about seven seconds, all the while taking deep, calm breaths. Gradually, he was to release the pressure, and, without detaching his finger from the point, he was to repeat the procedure at least five times. He should apply pressure to this point several times a day - morning, noon and evening - and because it was very accessible, he could easily do it at work or in any other place. This point was extremely important for him, since besides relieving the symptoms of his mid-life crisis, it was one of the optimal points for relieving tension, stress, and anxiety.

The second point was the pressure point on the sole of the foot [15]: Todd was to apply pressure to both feet alternately, beginning with his left foot. He would place his thumb on the point and apply gradual pressure, keep his thumb on the point for about ten seconds, and then gradually release the pressure, without taking his thumb off the point. He was to repeat the procedure three times. Then he had to repeat the whole thing on his right foot. This series of pressures was to be performed three times on each foot.

Todd was to practice applying pressure to the next two points both on a daily basis and before having intercourse. The first of these points was the "Original Chi" point [3], which is located in the center of the abdomen. He had to apply pressure gradually to this point with his thumb or with his forefinger. It was important for Todd not to release his finger from the point quickly, but to release the pressure slowly and gradually. He was to keep his finger on the point for about ten seconds, while taking deep breaths that reached right down into his abdomen. After the gradual release of the pressure, he was to repeat the procedure without lifting the finger from the point at all. This had to be done five times a day for the first months, and three times a day for the following months.

The second of these points was the "Walking Three Miles" point [4]: Todd was to apply pressure to the point in the same way as described above for the "Original Chi" point, but preferably three times a day, since this point was a very important one, which, besides helping to relieve Todd's mid-life crisis, would also help him generally fortify his body and soul.

Todd had to focus on the two above mentioned points for relieving tension and agitation. He was to practice applying these pressures on a daily basis. It was also extremely important for him to do it before he planned to have sex. Applying pressure to these points would help him to be relaxed, calm, and involved in his pleasure during sex, and would gradually help him liberate himself from the tension and anxiety that plagued his previous attempts at intercourse.

In addition, I recommended that Todd apply pressure to the following points in every situation in which he felt agitated, anxious, tense or worried. (These pressures would also help alleviate his tendency toward slightly higher-than-average blood pressure). The points were:

The point on the outer side of the calf [11]: Todd had to start with extremely gentle pressure, since this region was liable to hurt a bit when pressed because of his state of constant tension and cumulative imbalance. He could gradually increase the strength of the pressure on the point. He was to apply pressure gradually, keep his finger on the point for about seven seconds, and then release the pressure gradually. This procedure was to be repeated three times, and then Todd had to perform it on his other leg. Todd was told to begin with his left leg, and then move on to his right leg.

The second point was the pressure point between the upper lip and the nose [24]: Todd was to apply gentle pressure gradually to this point, using his forefinger or middle finger; the pressure must not be too strong. He had to repeat this procedure of applying and releasing pressure gradually at least three times, without detaching his finger from the point. While pressing, Todd was to take deep, slow, calm breaths. This pressure point is very easily accessible, so that Todd was advised to apply pressure to it each time he felt tense, stressed, worried or anxious - even at work or in a traffic jam. There is no limit to the number of times pressure can be applied to this point. It was important that Todd apply pressure to these two points especially when he got up in the morning and before he went to sleep at night. Before planning to have sex, he was to spend a few moments applying pressure to these points while lying on his back, in a calm, relaxed state, taking deep, calm, breaths, and relaxing his body.

After focusing on the second of the factors that were undermining Todd's sexual performance, we focused on strengthening his vitality and on arousing his sexual urge. To this end, Todd was to add pressure to the distant points to the series of pressures for treating sexual problems. He had to practice applying these pressures every day in order to increase his sexual potency, and integrate them into sexual intercourse, too.

The first point is the pressure point on the hand [22]: Todd was to apply "pinching" pressure to this point. Since he felt pain when this point was pressed during an examination that was performed on him, and this was an indication of a state of general imbalance in his body, he would have to begin with gentle pressure on this point, applied gradually, and then increased, until the pain gradually diminished. He was to apply the pressure to both hands, starting by applying gradual pressure to the left hand, keeping the finger on the point for five to ten seconds, at least three times on each hand. Todd was advised do it at other times during the day as well, when he had time.

The second point in this group was the point at the base of the calf [10]: Todd could apply pressure to this point with his thumb, or use the "pinching" technique, when most of the pressure is applied by the thumb that is placed on the point, and the rest of the fingers serve as supports.

Other points which Todd was advised to press on a daily basis were the points on the ear lobe [21] - gentle pressure on the part of the lobe that is parallel to the temple, keeping the finger on the point for five to seven seconds, and gradually releasing the pressure. Then, without detaching the finger from the point, the pressure on the point is gradually increased again, and this procedure is repeated three times. This was to be done two to three times a day.

While Todd was resting, taking a shower, or going to sleep, he was told to practice applying pressure to the points located on the five points (excluding the perineal point) of the "Conception Vessel" meridian [8]. These points are extremely important for fortifying and balancing the entire sexual system. Todd was to apply pressure to them with his thumb, or with his forefinger reinforced with his middle finger in order to increase the pressure. The pressures had to be steady, deep and slow, and Todd was to breathe regularly, slowly and deeply, right into his abdomen. He had to hold his finger on each point for about seven seconds, and repeat the procedure three to five times.

In addition to these pressure points, which Todd was told to work on every day regardless of actual intercourse, it was recommended that he and Jodi apply pressure to the Shiatsu for Lovers points that arouse sexual passion, and integrate them into foreplay and actual love-making. The points that arouse sexual passion are spread over four main areas: the back, the upper thigh, the perineum (the lower abdomen), and the ear, and besides being excellent arousal points during intercourse, they also reinforce sexual vigor, and contribute to fuller and better sexual functioning.

When Todd and Jodi wanted to have sex, they were advised to do the following in order to rehabilitate their sexual relations generally, and Todd's potency in particular.

First of all, they were not to start directly with intercourse, but rather use the various methods of arousal - even before foreplay. It was vital for Todd to distract his thoughts completely from the subject of whether he would have an erection or not, since this question created unnecessary anxiety, and undermined his sexual performance. It was very important that he perceive the sexual experience as a full, multifaceted experience, and enjoy every touch and every moment, allowing things to happen by themselves, and ridding himself of all his fears and anxieties. Before the couple had sex, Todd was to rest for an hour or more, so that he could be fresh, relaxed and free of daily cares that were certainly not helpful in his attempts to have an erection.

After this rest, the couple was to spend some time taking a warm, pleasant bath together, preferably with a mixture of essential oils such as jasmine, patchouli, sandalwood or cedarwood. Seven or eight drops of oil are sufficient for a bath that is filled with warm water, and they should be mixed gently into the bath-water.

When the couple were in the bath, they were to arouse each other naturally, by applying pressures in the following regions (with which they were already familiar): the inner and frontal regions of the thighs; the point on the outer side of the calf; the "Pass Organ" point, which is located in the center of the abdomen; the "Middle Extreme" point, which is located in the center of the slope of the abdomen; and the "Crooked Bone" point. Special attention was to be paid to the perineal point, located between the genitals and the anus. Contact with these points could include the application of pressures, caresses, and other forms of touch, taking note of the form of touch that was the most arousing for the partner.

After a long bath, which is both relaxing and sexually arousing, Todd and Jodi were to dry each other slowly and enjoyably, concentrating on the above mentioned points. After drying, the couple could rub each other with massage oil (some kind of vegetable oil, such as grape seed, almond or peanut oil, to which two or three drops of one of the previously mentioned essential oils are added). They could rub in the oil in bed, as part of a slow, pleasurable massage, focusing on the arousal points, as well as on the whole body and the sexual regions. It was very important for them to concentrate on the lower back region [19], since it contains numerous nerves that supply energy to the reproductive organs and control many vital functions of the lower body, among them erection and copulation. Fairly strong pressure was to be applied with the whole hand (because of Todd's full physical build), focusing on the regions on each side of the spinal column, right next to the vertebrae, but not on them, from slightly below the waist until above the tip of the tailbone.

After concentrating on these points, the points on the upper thigh were to be reached, using a slow, erotic, and pleasurable massage. These points are located on the front of the thighs. The massage should be performed using gentle pressure on the inner and frontal region of the thighs - a slow, gentle massage of the region, caresses, and arousing, stimulating touches of various kinds.

Obviously, Shiatsu for Lovers is a two-sided technique, with Todd giving it to Jodi, and Jodi giving it to Todd, while they constantly switched roles.

During the massage, desire should increase, as should sexual passion. A lot of time should be devoted to caresses, kisses, hugs and touch, as well as different forms of touch on the outer ear, such as nibbles, kissing, sucking the lobe, and so on. On the ear, there are important points for sexual arousal and increased desire, and they should not be ignored. It is also good to include pressures on the part of the ear lobe that is parallel to the temple - a very effective point in cases of impaired sexual function and sexual disorders, and for increasing sexual desire.

Gradually, the couple once more reached the "Love Points" - the points close to the genitals, that are extremely effective in improving sexual function and strengthening both male and female potency. Touching, pressing, and massaging these points would almost certainly lead to Todd's total arousal, since their action in this field is very significant. The "Pass Organ" point [5] is located in the center of the abdomen, below the navel. Gentle pressure should be applied to it, and it should be massaged and touched in various pleasurable ways. The "Middle Extreme" point [6] is located in the center of the slope of the abdomen, above the pubic bone, and the "Crooked Bone" point [7] is located at a distance of two finger-widths above the "Middle Extreme" point. These create a similar effect of arousal via pressure and massage. Now that it was very likely that Todd was feeling very sexually aroused, and would have an erection, there was no need to hurry, but rather to delay the passion a bit in order to increase it.

He and Jodi were now to focus on applying pressures to each other's "Conception Vessel" points [8]. After the pressure, massage and caressing of these points, the perineal point should be reached, and gentle pressure, alternating with caresses and various types of touch, should be applied with the finger. (See comment on page 62.)

At this point, if Todd persevered with his daily practice

sessions, there was a good chance that he would have a partial or full erection. He had to remember to be patient, and to recognize the added value of sexual intercourse and the overall enjoyment that he derived from it, while keeping his mind off the erection itself.

Todd and Jodi practiced Shiatsu for Lovers down to the last detail. During the first month, Todd reported that he still hadn't reached a full erection, but had achieved a partial one after only two weeks. However, he reported a significant improvement in his mood, as well as greater serenity and relaxation during the day, and he felt more alert and energetic. He felt that it was easier for him to free himself of the tensions and worries that plagued him frequently. Although he had not yet reached a full erection, he reported that his enjoyment of sex had increased enormously.

After less than three months of constant practice in applying Shiatsu pressures, he succeeded in achieving a full erection, and in enjoying full, satisfying sexual intercourse.

Although they accomplished their "objective," Todd and Jodi did not stop practicing the pressures. Jodi, who discovered the pleasure and the value of the pressures in raising her general vitality, as well as her sexual vitality and activity, also began to apply the pressures on a daily basis. Since she also received massage and pressure on her arousal points during foreplay, Jodi reached a much higher level of sexual satisfaction and orgasmic experiences than she had ever known. In an easy, simple, effortless and inexpensive way, Todd and Jodi succeeded in improving their sexual relations - and, as a result, their whole married life - and greatly increasing their enjoyment of and satisfaction from sexual intercourse.

Loss of libido as a result
of quitting smoking

Pamela, a 28-year-old single woman, resorted to Shiatsu for Lovers as a result of a loss of libido and functional problems during sexual intercourse. For many years, Pamela had derived a great deal of pleasure from intercourse, and was easily satisfied. She noted that her relationship with her boyfriend of two years' standing was pleasant and satisfying, and they enjoyed wonderful sexual compatibility.

Pamela was able to pinpoint exactly when her problem had begun. She had smoked since she was 18, and until recently, had been in the habit of smoking two packs a day. After she quit smoking, a few months previously, she began to experience disturbing and inexplicable agitation. She became hypersensitive, irascible and irritable, but since she did not permit herself to vent her anger at work or at home, she bottled it up inside, where it gnawed away at her. Since there had been no other changes in her life other than quitting smoking, it was clear to her that quitting smoking, as well as the urgent craving for the nicotine to which she had been addicted for so many years, were the causes of her agitation and feeling of lack that she experienced so frequently. Pamela declared that she was not prepared to use any form of medicinal tranquilizers or nicotine substitutes, and felt that she could get through this tiresome period, until her body and soul were totally free of the need for nicotine.

The thing that really bothered her enormously, however, was the loss of libido that she had experienced recently. Pamela described her feeling:

"When I get home from work in the afternoon, I'm already exhausted from the inner struggle with the agitation that I feel, and from the need to be on my guard all the time, so as not to light up a cigarette. I eat quickly, and go take a nap for a couple of hours. When Greg gets home, we go out, although now, because of my nervous state, we go out less than we did before, or we stay at home. At a certain point, the moment arrives when we get into bed. Although Greg tries to calm me down mentally and physically, I just can't shake off the tension. In the past, it was enough for him just to touch me for me to be immediately interested and turned on. Now, I often don't feel like getting into bed and having sex at all; I feel that I just don't have the patience for the whole thing. It bothers me, because ultimately, I always enjoyed sex a lot, especially with Greg, my present boyfriend. It never happened that I didn't desire him - unless I didn't feel well.

"After foreplay, when we reach the act itself, I often don't feel ready for intercourse, although the foreplay might have gone on for a long time. I feel far less turned on than in the past, and sometimes I just feel like getting the whole thing over with and going to sleep. I never used to have any trouble reaching orgasm, but now I often have that problem. That makes me even more agitated, because I'm aware that sexual satisfaction always relaxes me and makes me feel good. In fact, in the past, I would feel very energetic after intercourse.

"What's happening now is that instead of getting enjoyment and relaxation from sex, and experiencing the calmness and release that would help me get rid of the tension, I feel even more agitated because I didn't reach orgasm. The whole business of having sex has begun to be an annoying nuisance for me. I'd like to find a way to calm down in general, and more especially to restore my libido and my enjoyment of sex. I know that if there were any kind of technique that could help, Greg would be more than willing to cooperate."

It was recommended that Pamela and Greg try the following techniques:

First of all, Pamela had to apply pressure to three points on a daily basis:

The pressure point between the eyebrows [23]: Pamela had to try to apply pressure to this point every time she felt her agitation growing, as well as after washing her face when she got up in the morning, and before going to sleep at night. She was to apply gradual pressure to the point, pressing and releasing gradually, without detaching her finger from the point, five to seven times per session. Pressure on this point would help Pamela dispel some of the tension, agitation and stress from which she suffered most of the day.

The pressure point between the upper lip and the nose [24]: Pamela was told to apply gentle pressure to this point, pressing and releasing gradually, without detaching her finger from the point, at least five times per session. While applying pressure, she was to inhale and fill her chest cavity calmly, without effort, and exhale slowly while gradually releasing the pressure on the point. She was to apply pressure to this point every time she felt an increase in stress and tension, as well as in the morning and before going to sleep.

The point on the outer side of the calf [11]: Pamela was advised to apply pressure to this point at least three times a day, pressing and releasing gradually, without detaching her finger from the point. This procedure was to be repeated at least three times per session, while Pamela kept her finger on the point for at least seven seconds every time, making sure to take deep, calm breaths. At the beginning, pressure on this point was to be gentle, because it could be slightly painful as a result of the state of tension and agitation she was in.

Gradually, as the stress and tension decreased as a result of the daily pressure on the point, she would experience less pain, and then she could increase the strength of the pressure.

As for sexual intercourse: A half-hour to an hour before she planned to have sex, Pamela was to rest for a while, then get into a warm bath in which she mixed five to ten drops of lavender, neroli or patchouli oil, and stay there for 15 to 20 minutes. After drying herself off lightly, she was told lie on her back on the bed, and apply pressure to the three points described above, making sure to take deep, slow, calm breaths, and paying attention to her physical sensations.

When she had spent some time releasing the tensions by applying pressure to the points, Greg was to perform a slow, pleasurable massage on her in order to release tensions and as a preparation for the actual love-making, preferably using almond or grape seed oil mixed with two or three drops of neroli, lavender or patchouli oil.

During the massage, Greg was to focus on the following points: The pressure points on the lower back [19], to which he would apply gentle to medium pressure, using all the fingers in the regions on both sides of the spinal column.

By applying pressure to these regions, it is possible to help sexual arousal and increase Pamela's desire. Because of the proximity of these points to the genitals, and the relatively rapid effect that applying pressure to them has on increasing sexual desire, it was a good idea to incorporate the couple's favorite foreplay techniques into this stage.

During foreplay, several kinds of touch could be applied to the ear [21]: nibbles, kissing, sucking the lobe, and pressing the part of the lobe that is parallel to the temple - since touching these points causes sexual arousal and increased desire and passion during intercourse.

Both Pamela and Greg had to be very aware of their bodies, and be patient. Pamela was required to be aware of her level of arousal, and give herself the time to be sexually stimulated and aroused, without rushing ahead to perform intercourse as quickly as possible; in this way, she could experience the pleasure fully.

The next stage was applying pressure to the "Hui Yin" point (the perineal point), which is one of the most important points for erotic stimulation and sexual arousal. This point is located between the genitals and the anus. After applying gentle pressure several times to this point, pressure must be applied to the rest of the "Conception Vessel" points. The points are extremely important for sexual arousal, and when used in foreplay, they contribute significantly to increasing the stimulus both before and during intercourse.

It was very important for Pamela to be in tune with her feelings, both physical and psychological, and not rush into intercourse before she was ready. Greg had to be patient, and encourage her - even stopping the love-making if she did not feel relaxed or ready - knowing that what was good for her would be good for him, too!

Pamela and Greg practiced Shiatsu for Lovers for some time, and Pamela made sure to apply pressure to the points for releasing tension throughout during the day. She even made time for herself during work to practice applying pressure. Since most of the stress, just like her loss of libido, resulted from her quitting smoking, a situation that is neither terribly complicated nor protracted, she saw results almost immediately. First of all, the tension, agitation, and stress that she felt on a daily basis, were relieved to a great extent. Shortly after starting the Shiatsu practice, Pamela felt that she was getting back to her old self - where she was passionate, and enjoyed sex to the full. The removal of the barrier of stress and tension expressed itself immediately in her sex life.

To the joy of both partners, they discovered that, as a result of the Shiatsu for Lovers, especially during foreplay, not only did Pamela's sexual vigor return in full force, but they also achieved new heights of pleasure that they had not known before.

Even after Pamela's quitting smoking no longer bothered her, she and Greg continued to include the Shiatsu for Lovers in their sex lives, all the while discovering new, enjoyable and pleasurable ways of achieving even greater satisfaction. Both of them felt a great improvement in their level of desire and sexual arousal, as well as in the intensity of their orgasms, which became a sensual feast.

Shiatsu for Lovers during menopause

Michelle, a 45-year-old homemaker and mother of four children, told me about a disturbing problem that is extremely common among women in that age-group. Michelle, who was on the threshold of menopause, was suffering from the many symptoms that accompany this stage of life. While her periods had not yet entirely ceased, she suffered from irregularity and from tiresome menstrual pains. The hot flashes that had begun to bother her every now and then caused her not only physical discomfort, but embarrassment, especially when her face turned crimson while she was in company. Moreover, she was beginning to feel occasional mood swings She was more sensitive than ever before, and even the most trifling things caused her to burst into tears. During the day, she experienced occurrences of energy drain. She was also bothered by attacks of depression.

From the psychological point of view, she was greatly disturbed by the changes taking place in her body. As if these symptoms were not enough, her libido, which had always been steady and normal, had begun to decrease, creating a vicious circle that contributed to her feeling that she was becoming "less feminine and less sexy." The gradual decline in her libido caused an additional problem: Her husband, Ray, who himself was going through a mid-life crisis, was experiencing an increase in sexual desire, and was very keen to have sex more frequently than before. This situation created friction between Michelle and Ray, since Michelle preferred to go to sleep without having sex, while Ray wanted to have sex every night, and felt, on his part, that Michelle didn't desire him; he interpreted her unwillingness to have sex as withholding love and warmth from him.

When Michelle arrived for treatment, it was recommended

that she use Shiatsu for Lovers for soothing and alleviating her menopausal symptoms, and for increasing and arousing her sexual desire. In order to provide the couple with an additional dimension of psychological and physical proximity, it was suggested to Michelle that she and Ray apply the Shiatsu pressures to each other.

For daily practice, she was told to start off with a series of pressures on the points for relieving menopausal symptoms: the point that is located at the top of the nose [14], and the point that is located on the foot [15]. She was told to apply pressure to each of these points three times a day, and in each of these sessions, to apply pressure to each point three times.

In addition, because of her problems with painful, irregular periods, it was recommended that she practice applying pressure for the relief of menstrual cramps and pains on the point that is located below the knee [9], and on the point at the base of the calf [10]. Michelle applied the pressures for two weeks, and only saw the faintest results. Other points to help relieve her menopausal symptoms had to be added.

It was recommended that she add the "Intersection of the Three Yins" point [1] to her daily practice, using the "pinching" technique, three times a day. In addition, she had to apply pressure to the "Original Chi" point [3], which is located in the center of the abdomen, to the "Walking Three Miles" point [4], and to the "Sea of Blood" point [2] (Michelle was to recruit Ray's assistance for these last two points). Although the practice included many points, Michelle was also to add the pressure point at the outer side of the thigh [13], and Ray could help her with that one, too.

At first, Michelle was put off by the large number of

points to which she had to apply pressure every day. However, it was Ray who encouraged her to continue her daily practice. At first, because of Michelle's low energy level most of the day, she did not always feel like making the effort. Her frequent mood swings and her feelings of weakness were somewhat detrimental to the enterprise. Ray wouldn't give in, however, and he offered to apply pressure even to those points that Michelle could easily have pressed herself. Pressure was applied to the points every day; Ray's huge motivation created a good feeling of closeness and mutuality in her. The contact between them also contributed to their closeness, patience, and understanding.

There were prompt results. Michelle's hot flashes gradually became shorter and easier, and she no longer turned red in the face. While her periods never became regular, they were no longer painful, and Michelle got through them very easily. Her level of vitality improved beyond all recognition, and her mood swings became rarer, less extreme, and more fleeting. Her uncontrollable crying fits disappeared almost entirely.

Even her libido, which had decreased enormously because of all the menopausal symptoms, began to revive and balance itself. There is no doubt that the closeness and cooperation between Michelle and Ray contributed greatly to the improvement in her condition.

Because of the successful application of the pressure, and her revived energy, Michelle herself suggested to Ray that they use Shiatsu for Lovers for improving their sex life. Together they learned the points that arouse and strengthen the libido and the sexual system, and gradually they began to introduce them into their bedroom. Michelle began to realize that now, with her children leaving home, she and Ray had a lot more free time, and this could be a springboard for indulging in new activities and fulfilling wishes that she had never managed to fulfill in the past, because of a shortage of time and energy.

The couple began to take trips around the country, power-walk around their neighborhood every day, and, best of all, experience a renewed blossoming of their sex life. This, together with the new discoveries and excitement that the introduction of Shiatsu for Lovers into their sex life had yielded, plus the fact that they had more time for themselves, made their married life better, stronger, and more rewarding.

Lack of sexual satisfaction

Although Carly, a 25-year-old woman, had an active sex life, she did not find it very satisfying. While she reached orgasm, she felt that it did not satisfy her sufficiently. Years previously, she had had one sexual encounter in which she had experienced an incredible orgasm, but now she felt that her sexual enjoyment didn't come anywhere near the dizzying sensations that she had experienced during that one particular sexual encounter. Although she generally enjoyed the closeness and the love between her and her boyfriend, as well as the foreplay, her orgasm was very weak - just a slightly higher degree of arousal than the rest of the overall sexual experience.

Although she and her partner tried additional methods of sexual stimulation and arousal, as well as a variety of positions that might increase Carly's orgasmic pleasure, nothing changed. Moreover, it bothered her that it took her a long time to reach orgasm. Sometimes she would be very aroused right at the beginning of their love-making, but this arousal quickly waned, and she would need a very long period of foreplay - sometimes over an hour - until she felt aroused and ready for actual intercourse. This situation frustrated her, but she had resigned herself to it long since, because she did not know of any other way to increase the intensity of her orgasm and to experience quicker and more powerful sexual arousal.

After she came across the possibilities offered by Shiatsu for Lovers, Carly decided to apply pressure to several points, maintaining that "even if it doesn't help, it certainly won't hurt." At first, she focused on working on herself.

The points that she chose to press during the first stages were: the points on her ear [21]; the pressure point on her hand [22]; the point on the outer side of her calf, which is located at a distance of about three finger-widths below her kneecap, toward the outer side of her calf [11]; and the point at the base of her calf, which is located on the inner side of her leg [10]. She chose these points because of the ease with which she could apply pressure to them, and because they seemed very simple to begin with.

After about two weeks of daily application of pressure, she felt a certain degree of improvement in her general state of vitality, and there was a slight but discernible change in her capacity to be sexually aroused. During foreplay, she felt that she was aroused more easily, and although she had not yet felt an appreciable change in the intensity of her orgasm, the change in the strength of her arousal and in the degree of desire that she felt during foreplay contributed to the increase in her overall pleasure from love-making. Once she had experienced the good - though not yet sufficient - results that Shiatsu had yielded, she decided to apply pressure to additional points, and to have her partner participate in the procedure by asking him to press some of the points during foreplay.

On a daily basis, she added the points for the treatment of frigidity. Although Carly herself did not suffer from frigidity, she was correct in her choice - firstly because these points help to increase the libido and sexual arousal to a great extent, preventing it from waning after the initial arousal, and even increasing the intensity of the orgasm; and secondly, because frigidity is a variable concept, and only the woman herself can define her feeling. If she feels unsatisfied and unstimulated, and her orgasm is weak and insignificant, the Shiatsu for Lovers points described below are a good choice for her.

Carly began to work on the points of the stomach meridian on a daily basis. These points are located next to the region of the pubic bone [16]. She also worked on a point located below the knee [9]; on the points of the liver meridian, which are situated next to the thigh [17]; on the points of the spleen meridian, which are located on the inner part of the leg, next to the knee; and on a point above the ankle [18]. Moreover, she added the points on the front part of the thighs [20], which, besides increasing desire and reinforcing sexual vigor, strengthen the vitality of the whole body. Since this is a very large number of points, Carly stimulated them by pressure and massage of the inner and frontal region of the thighs.

Besides her daily practice, which she did alone, she told her partner about these points, and asked him to stimulate them during foreplay and love-making by caressing, massaging and pressing them. She also asked him to focus on the "distant" points for treating sexual problems, and to help her apply the daily pressure to these points, which improve all aspects of sexual function, increase the libido and sexual vigor, fortify the whole body, and improve its function.

Her partner learned the diagram of points on the back [19], and applied pressure with the pads of his hand, while Carly lay on the floor. He sat beside her, channeling the weight of his body into the root of the hand that was placed on the points. (Certain points were stimulated by direct pressure of his thumb and forefinger.) During foreplay, in order to increase the intensity of the sexual experience, he applied the pressures in a manner that resembled massage, in which he included caresses and touch, in order to arouse Carly in a sexy and calming way. During foreplay and love-making, her partner also focused on the points located along the "Conception Vessel" meridian [8]. After Carly experienced the beneficial effects of the pressure on these points during love-making, she added them to her daily sessions in order to strengthen and balance her whole sexual system.

The daily Shiatsu sessions that Carly had undertaken, as well as the inclusion of the points in love-making and foreplay, became easier, and it didn't take long for her to feel the welcome change. Gradually she began to feel that her sexual arousal during foreplay was becoming more appreciable, and did not wane, as it had in the past; the level of stimulus was maintained, and even increased. Carly began to experience more and more significant orgasms, and sometimes even especially strong ones that were no less amazing than the one she had had long ago. The length of time spent on foreplay in order to arouse her sexual desire and passion decreased, and she reached the stage where she was very aroused and passionate within 20 minutes.

To her great surprise, when she applied some of the pressures to her partner both on a daily basis and during love-making, he also experienced wonderful changes in his sexual functioning, ranging from a prolonged erection to a much more intense orgasm.

Carly was thrilled when she gained an additional benefit that was previously unfamiliar to her: multiple orgasms, starting with a light orgasm and continuing through a series of increasingly intense orgasms one after the other. The experiences that she had as a result of using Shiatsu for Lovers caused her to persist in her daily sessions, and inspired her and her partner to explore and apply pressure to additional points. By applying pressure to the perineal point

("Conception Vessel One" point) [8], which is located between the genitals and the anus, both partners experienced significantly increased erotic stimulation, and they learned to use this point and integrate it in various ways, ranging from the application of pressure to arousal using the tongue, into all the stages of foreplay and intercourse. Carly's partner discovered that the stimulation of this point aroused him in a way that he had not known before, and felt that the quality of sex had improved immeasurably since discovering this point.

In her daily sessions, Carly added the "Love Points": the "Pass Organ" point [5], which is located in the center of the abdomen, below the navel; the "Middle Extreme" point [6], which is located in the center of the slope of the abdomen, above the pubic bone; and the "Crooked Bone" point [7], which is located at a distance of two finger-widths above the "Middle Extreme" point. Although Carly and her partner's sex life was already so satisfying and pleasurable, she was surprised to discover that those points contributed greatly to intensifying their sexual pleasure.

Carly felt that Shiatsu for Lovers had changed her life in many areas, not just sexually. (Of course, the achievement of complete and full sexual satisfaction certainly changed Carly's general feeling, since the lack of satisfaction that she had experienced in the past had made her feel nervous and depressed.) She felt more lively, more alert, and much more focused and relaxed - and these factors manifested themselves both in her work and in her personal life.

Premature ejaculation

Earl, a 26-year-old man, suffered from a problem that plagues numerous men. Earl was a handsome man and a successful hair-stylist, whose natural charisma, good looks and conversational talents attracted many women. Despite these advantages, however, he had one "minor" problem that ruined his success with the opposite sex.

Between the ages of 18 and 23, Earl had had a steady girlfriend; they had had their first sexual experience together. Naturally, he had been extremely nervous the first time he had had sex, since he had never "gone all the way" before; moreover, since his girlfriend was a virgin, she was afraid of the pain he might cause her - and this made him nervous. To top it all off, they were in her parents' home, and he felt very ill at ease. For these reasons, the first time he had sexual intercourse, he ejaculated very quickly - the whole act occurred at lightning speed. His girlfriend did not enjoy it in the least. This caused Earl great anguish, and he felt that because he had not satisfied her at all, he had not "done his duty as a man."

Earl's good friend, who was more experienced than Earl, tried to cheer him up by reassuring him that he would no doubt "perform" much better next time, and would succeed in satisfying his girl. But this wasn't the case. Every time Earl and his girl started engaging in sexual activity, his excitement was enormous - so much so that he sometimes even ejaculated prior to penetration. Although he tried to satisfy his girlfriend in other ways, he was unable to maintain foreplay for any length of time, since it intensified his excitement and diminished his chances of preventing premature ejaculation. It was a no-win situation, since the longer the foreplay continued, the more aroused and excited

Earl became, the more anxious he felt about his performance, and the quicker he ejaculated - sometimes without even penetrating.

Because of his anxiety and his disappointment in himself, he was not interested in renewing their sexual activity after he had ejaculated, and would withdraw into himself, feeling regret and remorse vis-a-vis his girlfriend, who had not been sexually satisfied. Unfortunately, because she was so young and inexperienced, she was unable to understand his predicament, and although she did not say it directly, she expressed her disappointment in his sexual performance in many other ways. Earl's feeling was, "If I can't satisfy my girl, what good am I?" In spite of the fact that he was a very sensual person by nature, sexual intercourse began to appear to him as an unpleasant experience involving a great deal of mental suffering. As a result, the frequency with which they had sex diminished.

When he reached the age of 23, his girlfriend met and fell in love with somebody else. Earl felt that her new lover was much less handsome and good-hearted than he was. He couldn't understand her attraction to the other guy, or why she had left Earl for him. The only obvious reason he could think of was that since he had been unable to satisfy her sexually, she had undoubtedly dumped him for someone else whose performance in the sack was better.

This dealt a serious blow to Earl's self-esteem, and from that time on, he made no effort to seek out female company. Because of his good looks, Earl was very sought after, but, deep in his heart, he considered the whole female sex to be threatening. He decided that every woman wanted to be satisfied in bed, and that was what was most important to her." For this reason, he refrained from accepting the many propositions that came his way.

When he occasionally agreed to go out with somebody, and they landed up in bed, the scenario would repeat itself. Even if the woman in bed with him understood him, and wanted to continue the relationship anyway, Earl was sure that she "just wanted to console him," and that there was no chance of anything serious developing between them after she had witnessed what he defined as "his pathetic performance in bed." He reached the conclusion that there was nothing more to be done - there was no way he could delay his ejaculation.

He began to shy away from the company of women. Girls he liked, and who tried to establish a deeper relationship with him, became "platonic friends." He took care not to go to bed with them, so that they wouldn't find out what a "lousy lover" he was, as he put it.

One of these women, who had become a close "platonic" friend, was an acupuncture and Shiatsu practitioner. She refused to accept his pessimistic assumption that there was no way the situation could be changed. It took a long time for her to convince him just to try applying pressure to a few points that were nowhere near his genitals. The eternal claim that "even if it doesn't help, it certainly won't hurt, and if you don't try it, you'll never know what you missed" ultimately got the better of Earl.

His friend placed a firm mattress on the floor, and told him to lie on his back. Since she understood that a large part of his problem stemmed from his inability to relax and remain somewhat "cool-headed" during sex, and she could discern slight agitation below the surface, she decided to focus first and foremost on points for relieving extreme tension, knowing that if he continued applying pressure himself on a daily basis, he would feel the beneficial effects of the Shiatsu pressures, and then it would be possible to teach him additional points.

While Earl was lying on the mattress, his friend applied pressure to the point located in the space between his eyebrows [23]. She told him to take deep breaths and relax his body, and used her forefinger to exert gentle pressure on the point. She applied pressure gradually, holding her finger on the point for about 10 seconds, and then gradually released the pressure. Without detaching her finger from the point, she repeated the procedure five times.

After the pressure on this point, Earl was calmer, and his friend went on to the next pressure point - the point between the upper lip and the nose [24]. Here too she applied gentle, gradual pressure with her forefinger, held her finger on the point for about 10 seconds, and then gradually released the pressure. She also repeated this procedure five times, while ensuring that Earl was taking deep, slow, calm breaths all the while.

After applying pressure to the two points mentioned above, Earl's friend concentrated on applying pressure to the point on the outer side of the calf [11]. In order to measure the distance, she measured Earl's fingers so that she could identify the precise location of the point. Because of Earl's ongoing state of imbalance, and his inner agitation, his friend applied the pressure very gently, since Shiatsu for Lovers is not meant to hurt in any way whatsoever.

Following this brief session, Earl felt very alert, relaxed and calm. His friend explained that, while the pressures were very simple, he had to start to apply pressure to the points on a daily basis in order to achieve far-reaching results. She advised him to apply pressure to the above mentioned points, or at least to the pressure point between the eyebrows and the one between the upper lip and the nose, whenever he felt any degree of agitation, tension, or anxiety (over and above the daily sessions). He should do so while working at the beauty parlor, during his leisure time, or after a long day of work or a great deal of pressure, so as to induce a state of calmness, relaxation, and release from the agitation that accompanied these situations. This would facilitate the psychological release from tension and anxiety so that he could function better. She explained to him that these points had proved themselves in improving sexual functioning; after daily sessions, he too would see positive results.

Earl still had trouble believing that such simple pressure points could solve his problem, but he began to practice, and enjoyed the resulting calmness and the higher level of vitality. He experienced great relief from the tension and agitation that had been an inextricable part of his life, and he was surprised to discover that after a week of practice, the headaches that had often bothered him at the end of the day began to decrease in intensity, and finally ceased.

At the end of two weeks of treatment, Earl's friend added some more pressure points - the "distant" points for treating sexual problems. The aim of these points was to improve every aspect of sexual functioning. These points, besides their beneficial effects in the field of sexual activity, have a varied and extremely significant effect, and fortify the entire body by increasing its vitality and balancing both the physical and psychological condition of the person.

These points - which also play a significant role during intercourse - contribute to the increase in sexual arousal. They demonstrate the advantage of Shiatsu for Lovers over conventional treatment of various kinds. Although they are supposed to arouse the person, they also relax him, by effecting the correct balance. When there is a need to "moderate" the degree of arousal, they do this just as effectively as they increase sexual arousal.

Earl's friend taught him to apply pressure to the point that is located on the gap between the thumb and the forefinger [22], and to the point at the base of the calf, which is located on the inner side of the leg, on the lowest part of the calf [10]. She added the "Intersection of the Three Yins" point [1], as well as the "Sea of Blood" point [2].

After the first points had been pressed for about two weeks, Earl's friend added the "Original Chi" point [3], as well as the "Walking Three Miles" point [4]. These points are known for their effect on the sexual system, and for balancing the sexual system according to the individual's need, and are also used for general strengthening and for increasing vitality.

Round about that time, Earl met a charming woman who captured his heart from the very first moment. For two months, despite the tremendous passion they felt for each other, Earl managed to avoid sexual intercourse. But at a certain stage, his new girlfriend began to wonder about his abstinence. She was free and open, and was not ashamed to admit to Earl that she desired him, and that it surprised her that he foiled all her attempts to have intercourse. As a result of the openness of their relationship, he shyly told his girlfriend about the problem he considered so earth-shattering. To his joy, she grasped the situation, and accepted it naturally. She was pleased to hear that he was using Shiatsu to solve the problem, and announced that she would be happy to learn to apply the pressure and try it with him, so that she too could help solve the problem. Her patience, and the way in which she had accepted his problem, stirred hope in Earl's heart.

It was the first time in almost two years that he agreed to have sexual intercourse. He asked his girlfriend to help him apply pressure to some of the points when they got into bed. In order to relieve the tension even more, Earl preferred to put off getting undressed for a bit, and his girlfriend applied the Shiatsu pressures, combining them with massage and pressing movements. The movements gradually became more sexual, until Earl felt free and liberated, and they flowed into slow, enjoyable sexual intercourse. To Earl's surprise, he held out for longer than he had in the past. His ejaculation still occurred quickly, but there was certainly an improvement. He was surprised, especially considering the fact that it was so long since he had had sex, and he was very turned on. He felt that despite the excitement he had experienced at the sight of his girlfriend's naked body, and the pleasurable sensations of the contact that had turned him on in the extreme, he was much calmer than before, more cool-headed, so that he could control his actions during love-making to a much greater extent, and give his girlfriend greater satisfaction.

Now that Earl had a loyal partner with whom to experiment and apply Shiatsu techniques, they both decided to try out additional pressure points. They added the pressure points along the "Conception Vessel" meridian [8] to their foreplay. The couple aroused each other by applying steady pressures and keeping their finger on each point for a few seconds, all the while combining the pressure with enjoyable and stimulating contact. They both experimented with the points on the inner and front parts of the thighs [20] in order to stimulate each other to a great extent, and

Earl's girlfriend discovered that these pressures, plus massage, caresses, and oral contact on the region, stimulated and aroused her, and made her passion soar to new heights. Touching and applying pressure to the perineal point [8] caused both of them to experience incredible sensations.

After a short time, Earl succeeded in achieving relatively far-reaching results. He managed to control his ejaculation for a long time, and even got to the point where he reached orgasm and ejaculated only after his girlfriend had had at least one orgasm, and sometimes even more. This delighted Earl, and made him feel like a man in a way that he had never felt before. He finally felt that the sexual tension that had plagued him for so long had been released.

The improvement that had occurred in his sex life affected every aspect of his life - from paying more attention to how he dressed to feeling more comfortable in his place of work, where he could now stand up for himself and get what he wanted with far more assertiveness. He felt as if his life had changed beyond recognition. His self-confidence increased in quantum leaps, and his creativity, which had long been repressed, began to flourish.

Problems of irregular periods and menstrual cramps

One of the advantages of Shiatsu for Lovers is that the pressure can be applied to young and old recipients alike. Sometimes, more than one member of the same family requires the application of Shiatsu pressure in order to improve his physical and mental functioning in general, and his sexual function in particular.

Merrill, a woman of 38, had suffered badly during her periods for many years. Every month, she spent the long days of her period in agony, reduced to a limp rag. She suffered from backaches, abdominal pains, dry, brittle, unmanageable hair that was impossible to style, as well as acute agitation, which was sometimes replaced by mild depression, during which the most minor things could upset her out of all proportion and cause her to be hypersensitive and tearful.

In addition to her suffering during her period, the days preceding it were no bed of roses, either. About five days before her period was due, Merrill would begin to experience the phenomena of agitation, insatiable hunger, an extreme craving for sweet things, and an increased appetite. The skin on her face and body tended to dry out during the premenstrual days, and all the symptoms together made her feel awful and depressed. After these miserable days, her period arrived, very heavy, and lasted for at least five days, sometimes even a whole week.

Merrill underwent gynecological and hormonal examinations, which did not reveal any specific problem. Her condition was defined as "normal," but none of this helped her on the days when she felt listless, nervous, sensitive, impatient, and sore.

Merrill's 14-year-old daughter, Vanessa, didn't have a great time during her periods, either. She had started menstruating at the age of 12, but in those two years, her periods had not yet become regular - either in the intervals at which they occurred, the length of time they lasted, or in the amount of bleeding, which differed from period to period. Moreover, Vanessa suffered from premenstrual pain in her breasts, and from severe back and abdominal pains during her period, which disrupted her daily activities at school, socially, and on trips.

After trying several methods of treatment that were not particularly effective, the two turned to Shiatsu for Lovers, which offers good and effective solutions for balancing the sexual and reproductive systems as well as the whole body (and not only for purposes of love-making and intercourse).

At first, both Merrill and Vanessa were offered similar treatment plans, including applying pressure to points for the relief of menstrual cramps and pains. The pressure point below the knee [9]: Vanessa was told to apply pressure to this point at least twice a day, while Merrill, whose problem had been going on for much longer, was told to apply pressure five times a day during the first week, and three times a day during the second week.

The pressure point located at the base of the calf [10]. Vanessa was advised to apply pressure to this point twice a day, while Merrill had to do so five times a day for the first two weeks, and three times a day in the third week. (It is preferable to use the "pinching" technique.)

The pressure point located above the knee [12]: Merrill and Vanessa were told to apply pressure to this point three times a day.

Another important point that they both had to work at was

the pressure point on the thigh [13], which is known to be extremely effective in relieving menstrual pains and cramps. It was recommended that Merrill and Vanessa help each other apply pressure to this point, while they were both standing; one was to apply pressure to the other with her spread hand placed at the base of the buttocks, and the pressure applied gradually to the point by the thumb, which remained on the point for about seven seconds, and was then gradually released. Without detaching the thumb from the point, Merrill and Vanessa had to repeat the procedure three times. Vanessa was to apply pressure to this point three times a week, while Merrill had to do so five times a week during the first two weeks, and three times a week after that.

Vanessa was told to apply pressure three times a week to some additional points two weeks after she had started pressing the points mentioned above, while Merrill had to start immediately, following the pressure on the first points, and she should make sure to do so every day, three times a day.

Applying pressure to these points is very effective, and even if the results are not immediately forthcoming, completion of the session will lead to extremely significant results.

These points include: The "Intersection of the Three Yins" point [1]: Gradual pressure should be applied to this point, keeping the finger on the point for 10 seconds, and then releasing the pressure gradually. Without detaching the thumb from the point, this procedure should be repeated.

Merrill and Vanessa were to help each other to apply pressure to the "Sea of Blood" point [2], with one sitting on a chair, and the other, seated on the floor (or on a cushion) in front of her, covering her kneecap with her hand. The point is located beneath the thumb of the "presser," and pressure should be applied to it gradually; then the thumb should be kept on the point for 10 seconds, followed by the gradual release of the pressure. Without detaching the thumb from the point, this procedure should be repeated at least three times.

The "Original Chi" point [3]: Merrill was to apply pressure gradually to this point with her thumb or forefinger, keeping the finger on the point for five to ten seconds, then gradually releasing the pressure. Without detaching the thumb from the point, this procedure should be repeated about three times.

The "Walking Three Miles" point [4]: Pressure was to be applied to this point when Merrill was sitting in an armchair, with Vanessa placing her hand on her kneecap. The point should be pressed with the thumb. The procedure of gradually applying and releasing pressure should be repeated at least three times.

This point is extremely important, since, alleviating menstrual pains and cramps, it is used for general strengthening and increasing the level of general vitality of the body. For this reason, Vanessa was also to apply pressure to this important point.

In order to achieve optimal, rapid and clear-cut results in the relief of menstrual pains, both Merrill and Vanessa had to make sure to apply pressure to the points regularly, making time for it - even during busy, stressful days. Since Merrill suffered for several days before her period, as well as during it, from severe and disturbing agitation, which disrupted her daily activities and influenced every area of her life, it was very important that she continue applying daily pressure to the points that relieve tension. The advantage of these points is their relatively rapid effect. Already during the first stages of applying pressure to them, results in the form of reduced daily stress were evident, as well as a feeling of calmness and tranquillity that lasted the entire day, even without any direct link to the agitation and hypersensitivity before and during the period. It is important to devote some time to applying pressure to the points on a daily basis, and not just when the irksome symptoms appear. After all, prevention is better than cure.

The points that were recommended to Merrill were: the point on the outer side of the calf [11], and the pressure point between the upper lip and the nose [24]. Pressure should be applied gradually to these points with the thumb or forefinger, and then released gradually. The last two points should be pressed gently, because of the sensitivity of their locations. Merrill was to apply light pressure to each one at least three times, holding her finger on the point for seven to ten seconds each time. Without detaching her finger from the point, she was to repeat the procedure. While applying pressure to the points, as well as to the pressure point between the upper lip and the nose and to the pressure point between the eyebrows, the manner of breathing is very important, as it adds to the immediate and cumulative effect of relaxation; for this reason, it was important for Merrill to take deep breaths while applying pressure.

Merrill and Vanessa meticulously followed the plan that had been prescribed for them. At first, the plan seemed "heavy" and difficult to apply, especially for Vanessa, because of the large number of pressure points. However, as they got into the swing of the daily sessions, they discovered that they took up very little time, and were easy to do. The first results that they experienced were in their daily activities, when they noticed that within a fortnight of starting to apply the pressures, there was an obvious improvement in their mood, in their ability to concentrate (a very significant factor for Vanessa, as a high-school student), in their alertness, and in their general level of vitality.

Their first period after they had begun applying the pressures was easier, but they both still felt pain and great discomfort. However, Merrill felt far less disturbed an agitated, even after such a short time, although she still had pain. During her second period after applying the pressures, Vanessa still had a slight backache and abdominal cramps, but they were relatively mild, and her mood was good during her entire period. She went to school and participated in all the activities, just like on any other day. Merrill noticed a significant difference in the intensity of her pains, as well as in the length of her period, which was now shorter than it used to be, with a far more normal volume of bleeding. She also functioned normally on those days, and although she was more sensitive than on regular days, she did not manifest this sensitivity outwardly.

Over time, by applying pressure to the points regularly, Merrill and Vanessa reached the stage that besides the normal inconvenience, nothing stopped them from doing their regular, everyday activities during the days preceding their period, and during the period itself. The pain that accompanied their periods gradually diminished, as did their mood swings, which became less noticeable. Merrill said that she still had a craving for sweet things a few days before her period, but now she was satisfied with two or three squares of chocolate, and the "bad old days" of uncontrolled eating gradually decreased until they disappeared altogether.

Even after they had experienced an appreciable improvement in their condition, and had accomplished their coveted objective, Merrill and Vanessa continued to apply pressure to the points regularly twice a week, both for maintaining the balance that had been achieved, and for the enjoyment and the feeling of calmness and energy that had come from applying pressure to Shiatsu points.

The problem of a low potential for pleasure and a weak sexual urge

Dana, a good-looking woman in her thirties, was introduced to Shiatsu for Lovers by a friend who had used the method herself and had given it a glowing report. The problem from which Dana was suffering was one that was common among men and women alike, but there is a tendency - possibly justified - to relate it more to women.

Dana suffered from a weak sexual urge, and from a very low potential for sexual pleasure. Sexual intercourse, which is undoubtedly one of life's pleasures, and an inextricable part of daily life and married life, simply "passed her by" without her experiencing a trace of pleasure or enjoyment.

Unfortunately, although this problem is so widespread, many women do not have it treated, simply because they have "gotten used" to the situation and resigned themselves to it, or because of a lack of awareness or knowledge of the pleasure that can be derived from sexual intercourse.

In Dana's case, all the relevant factors for enjoying satisfying sex like anyone else were normal. In spite of everything, though, the pleasure she derived from sex was so minimal as to be almost imperceptible. She didn't feel any real pleasure. During intercourse, and even during foreplay, she felt that she just "happened to be there," without any significant or satisfying stimulation.

The fact that she did not suffer from any physical disorder, and that all the processes that should occur in her body during intercourse did in fact occur - but despite everything, she had no enjoyment whatsoever - frustrated and depressed her. The constant lack of satisfaction was accompanied by additional symptoms, which were caused by it; Dana felt listless most of the time, and mildly depressed.

While the physical proximity of her husband - his kisses, embraces and caresses - fulfilled her need for warmth and physical closeness, she had gradually "trained" him to skip foreplay, which didn't give her any pleasure and just frustrated her, and get straight down to actual intercourse; she wouldn't enjoy it in any case, so "she might as well get it over with as quickly as possible."

One of Dana's good friends, to whom Dana confided her misery and frustration, had tried Shiatsu for Lovers in order to improve her weak and unsatisfying orgasms during intercourse. After she experienced a tremendous improvement, and saw fantastic results, she rushed to share her wonderful secret with Dana, and implored her to try just a few pressure points in order to extricate herself from the endlessly frustrating situation she was in. Dana was pleased with this suggestion, since after years of a lack of sexual satisfaction, she was ready to try anything that could change things.

She began to apply Shiatsu techniques on a daily basis, but was afraid to tell her husband about them, since she didn't know how much the application of pressure would help, and she didn't want to raise false hopes.

To start off with, Dana chose the points that are used to treat frigidity. Although she wasn't frigid, according to popular definition, she felt that these points could help her. She assiduously practiced applying pressure to the points of the stomach meridian [16], to the points of the liver meridian [17], and to the points of the spleen meridian [18]. She applied pressure to the points for two weeks, and after some time, she began to feel a tiny, but perceptible improvement. She did not know whether this improvement was genuine, or whether it was a psychological result of applying pressure to the points, but she decided to continue, and to add more points.

She added the "distant" points for dealing with sexual problems to her daily sessions, beginning with the point on the hand [22], because of its accessibility and the possibility of applying pressure to it easily wherever she was. She made sure to apply pressure to the previously mentioned points three times a day, and added the new point many times a day.

After some time, she added to her daily sessions the point that is located on the outer side of the calf [11], as well as the point at the base of the calf [10. She applied gradual pressure to these points, too, keeping her finger on the point for about 10 seconds, and then gradually releasing the pressure. She repeated the procedure on each point three times in each session.

The addition of these pressure points to her daily sessions was quick to produce clear-cut results, though not particularly for her original problem. Since these points have a variety of effects that fortify the entire body, Dana began to feel more energetic, more alert, less tired, and better-tempered. There were soon tangible results in the area of sex, too. To her great astonishment, she felt an increase in her general libido. Although she had not yet reached the coveted orgasm, she often felt that she really wanted to have intercourse, and her eagerness before and during sex increased enormously. During foreplay, too, she experienced new sensations, although they were still rather weak, but she had no doubt that there was a significant difference between her sensations before she started practicing the pressures, and after.

She now felt that she could tell her husband about the new

method she had tried in order to solve her problem. Actually, she didn't have much choice, since he had noticed the difference, and begged her to tell him what was happening in her life to cause such a transformation during sex. When he heard about the Shiatsu pressures, he got very excited, and asked her to keep it up. Dana requested that he help her apply the pressures. Now that foreplay was suddenly worth more to her, and she felt a genuine and strong desire to increase her sensations, she asked him to include some of the pressure points in their foreplay.

Dana added the "Love Points" to her daily sessions. These are the points that are located near the genitals, and they are extremely effective in improving sexual functioning and increasing sexual vigor and libido. She applied pressure three times a day to the "Pass Organ" point [5], to the "Middle Extreme" point [6], and to the "Crooked Bone" point [7].

When Dana and her husband included pressures on these points during foreplay and intercourse, they discovered that this aroused Dana in a way that she had never known before, and although she still had not reached orgasm, she began to derive enormous pleasure from sexual intercourse, and especially from foreplay. Sensations that had previously been unfamiliar to her, eagerness and passion that had never characterized her, began to stir inside her. Many times, she even felt that she was close to orgasm, and was hopeful that by means of Shiatsu for Lovers, which had already proved its effectiveness, she would also achieve orgasm.

Her sexual appetite increased unrecognizably, causing a renewed blossoming in her relationship with her husband. At the same time, she began to feel more sexy and attractive, and this was also evident in the change that took place in the way she dressed; she replaced her conservative wardrobe with more flattering and attractive clothes, and paid more attention to her general appearance.

Dana continued to apply Shiatsu pressures assiduously, but now she only did so about twice a day, adding the pressure point on the part of the ear lobe [21]. Since she felt that this point was of obvious help in increasing her libido, she asked her husband to focus on her ear during foreplay. She discovered that blowing, nibbling and licking her ear lobe aroused and stimulated her, and caused her to be more active and assertive during intercourse.

Gradually, together with her supportive and understanding husband, she added to her daily sessions the points for arousing sexual desire that are located on the back [19]. Her husband applied medium pressure with all his fingers to both sides of the spinal column. Once a day, he applied the pressures to her body, and before they got into bed, he applied the pressures to her naked body once more, while arousing her and sweeping her into passionate love-making.

While still applying pressure to the points and massaging Dana's back, when he felt her sexual arousal begin, he would gently turn her over onto her back and softly apply pressure to the "Pass Organ" point, to the "Middle Extreme" point, and to the "Crooked Bone" point. Then he would slowly reach the "Conception Vessel One" point [8], which is located between the genitals and the anus. He would stimulate it gently by alternating pressure and release. Pressure on this point literally drove Dana out of her mind, and turned her on wildly. But her husband knew that it was possible to increase her passion even more, and after arousing this point, he continued on to the next points on the

"Conception Vessel" meridian, which continue along the center line of the lower abdomen. Dana's husband stimulated them by applying steady pressure, and keeping his finger on each point for a few seconds, while he kissed and caressed Dana's body in order to prevent the pressures from become too "technical."

In addition, applying pressure to the points on the inner and front parts of the thighs [20] greatly stimulated Dana, especially when her husband alternated the pressures with massage, caresses, or nibbles in the region.

After the points on the thighs, Dana felt sufficiently hot and turned on to initiate the transition to intercourse herself.

The first time she reached orgasm, she was so surprised and excited that she almost cried. She had never believed that sex could provide such tremendous, vibrant pleasure.

By persisting in her daily sessions, the pleasure she derived from sex grew and increased, and today she enjoys a pleasurable and satisfying sex life in every way.

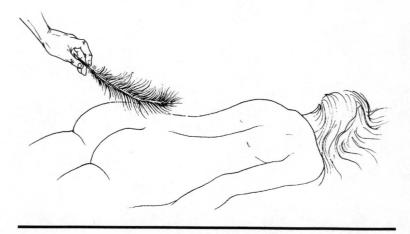